Cooking to Conceive

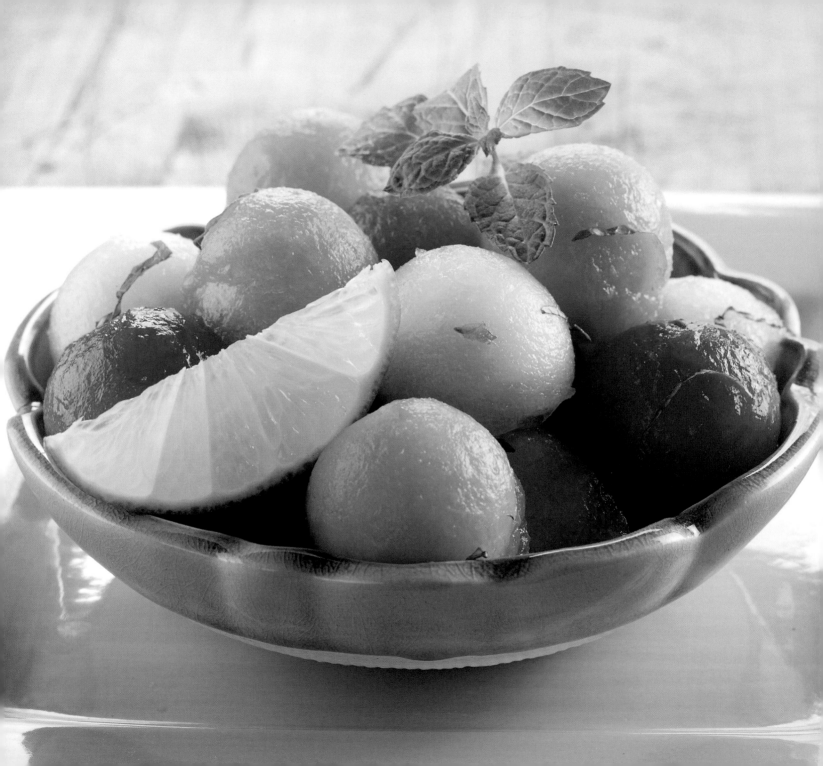

Cooking to Conceive

Fertility-Boosting Foods & Recipes to Help You Get Pregnant

By Kim Hahn and the Editors of *Conceive Magazine*
Foreword by Susan L. Treiser, M.D., Ph.D.

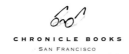

CHRONICLE BOOKS
SAN FRANCISCO

Library of Congress Cataloging-in-Publication Data available.
ISBN 978-0-8118-6854-9

Manufactured in China

Design by Patrick Greenish
Photography by Susan Bourgoin
Food Styling by Mary Holloway and Wendy Holloway
Indexed by Michelle Graye

Based on information published in *Conceive Magazine*: Founder, Kim Hahn; Editorial Director, Beth Weinhouse; Managing Editor, Emily Kruckemyer; Creative Director, Patrick Greenish.

10 9 8 7 6 5 4 3 2 1

www.conceiveonline.com

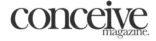

Chronicle Books LLC
680 Second Street
San Francisco, California 94107

www.chroniclebooks.com

ACKNOWLEDGMENTS

For this, *Conceive*'s third book project, there are several people we'd like to thank.

First and foremost, we want to thank Charity Ferreira for her culinary expertise, and for developing the recipes that fill these pages. At *Conceive* we know all about fertility, but we were very fortunate to be working with Charity, who knows all about food. We worked together for months to determine the mix of recipes that would fulfill all our requirements: certainly they had to contain fertility-boosting ingredients, but in addition they had to be easy to make, not require exotic ingredients, be the kinds of food that people eat every day, and, of course, taste delicious. Somehow Charity managed to work within these guidelines and satisfy all these requirements. We were very lucky to have her on board with us. A big thank you, too, to Charity's recipe tester, Kate Washington . . . who became pregnant while working on this book! (FYI, she credits the Pumpkin Macaroni and Cheese on page 96.)

Second, we'd like to thank Susan Bourgoin, our very talented food photographer. Susan and her staff prepared the recipes in this book, faithfully procuring ingredients and following instructions so that what you see on the page is what you can make at home. (And from trying samples at the photo studio we can attest that these recipes taste great.) Susan's excitement and flexibility made the project great fun. Thank you also to Susan's assistant, Susan Lindsay. And to Mary Holloway and her daughter Wendy, who were the stylists on the photo shoot and helped make our food as beautiful as it is tasty.

We're also indebted to Chronicle Books for their support, and this cookbook is *Conceive*'s third happy project with the publisher. Many thanks to our editor Ursula Cary, who inherited this book from a predecessor but saw its potential and got us all through our first cookbook project.

Finally, we'd like to thank the many writers who have contributed to *Conceive Magazine* since its inception in 2004. They helped report and present the information on nutrition and fertility that was first published in *Conceive* and that now forms the basis for this cookbook.

TABLE OF CONTENTS

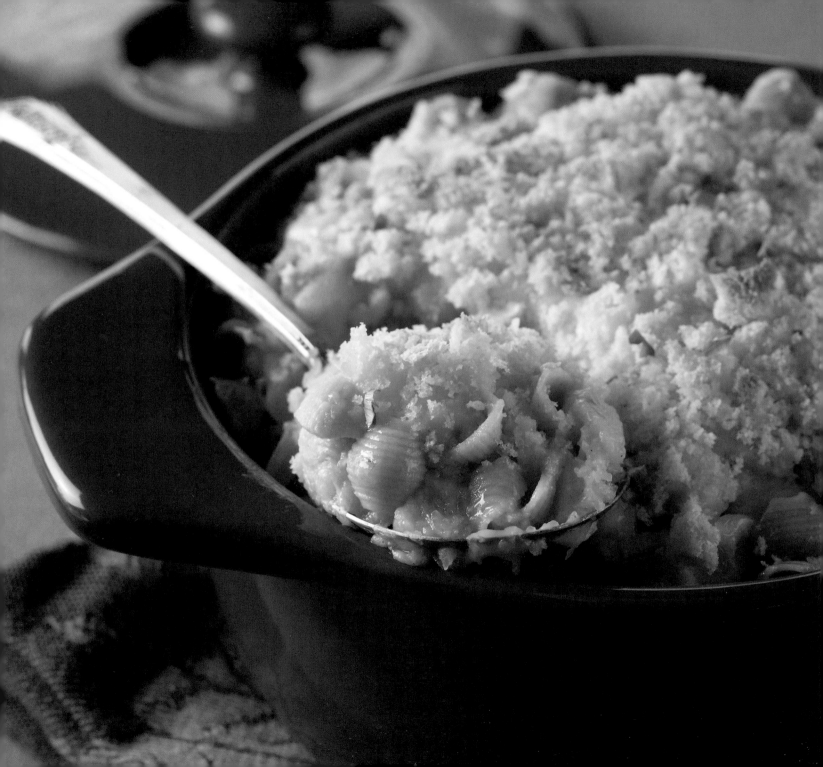

FOREWORD

As a physician specializing in fertility treatment for the last twenty years, I'm often surprised by how much my patients know about their reproductive health . . . and how much they don't.

In particular, I find that people don't realize how much their lifestyle choices can affect their fertility. Cigarette smoking, for instance, can lower sperm quality for men and make it more difficult for women to conceive. Certain medications can be harmful, as can recreational drugs.

One of the factors that plays a major role in reproductive health is diet. Our nutrition and weight can have a big influence on our capacity to conceive and carry a healthy pregnancy. It really shouldn't be a surprise. Just as wise food choices can help prevent diabetes and heart disease, eating healthy and maintaining an optimal weight can help keep women's and men's bodies primed for procreation. Choosing the "right" proteins, fats, vitamins, and minerals can keep men's and women's reproductive systems functioning at their healthy best.

In the fertility clinic where I work as a reproductive endocrinologist, I see patients every day who have tried without success to conceive naturally. These couples are looking for a medical solution to help them have a baby. Since my goal is to help couples become parents, I wish more people were aware of their reproductive health and how their lifestyle choices can affect it before they need to resort to medical treatment.

Obviously not all fertility issues can be overcome with lifestyle choices, and many are beyond an individual's control. But getting the right nutrients to keep hormone levels and reproductive organs healthy is smart at any age and any stage, before trying to conceive, while trying, and during pregnancy. The opening pages of this cookbook clearly and accurately explain the science of nutrition as it applies to fertility, and how people hoping to become parents can make their daily diets an ally in their quest for parenthood.

Cooking to Conceive is filled with delicious, simple-to-prepare recipes that make eating to get pregnant fast and fun. The foods are the kinds of things that most of us eat regularly, altered a bit to maximize their fertility-boosting ingredients. There are recipes for morning, noon, and night, snacks, and even suggestions for meals to get couples in the mood for love (and baby making). The recipes are delicious and wholesome, and they even can be served to guests, who'll never suspect the hidden benefits (don't worry, no one can get pregnant just by eating these foods!).

Conceive Magazine entered the national market in 2004, with groundbreaking information and articles for women who hoped to become pregnant. The magazine has experienced phenomenal success, and I am honored to have been a regular columnist (Consulting Room) as well as a member of the advisory board.

No national publication of its kind existed prior to *Conceive*, and it has filled a long overlooked niche in the marketplace.

Over the last few years, *Conceive* has proved to be a destination publication for couples searching for advice, answers, and qualified professional information and opinions regarding fertility. A vast scope of interesting articles and support are offered in every issue both in print and online.

Cooking to Conceive is an excellent collection of everyday recipes that any couple can incorporate into their regular routine to improve health in general, and fertility health in particular. This book, the third produced by Kim Hahn and the editors of *Conceive*, is another excellent choice for anyone contemplating parenthood.

Bon appetit!

Susan L. Treiser, M.D., Ph.D.
Cofounder and Codirector
IVF New Jersey

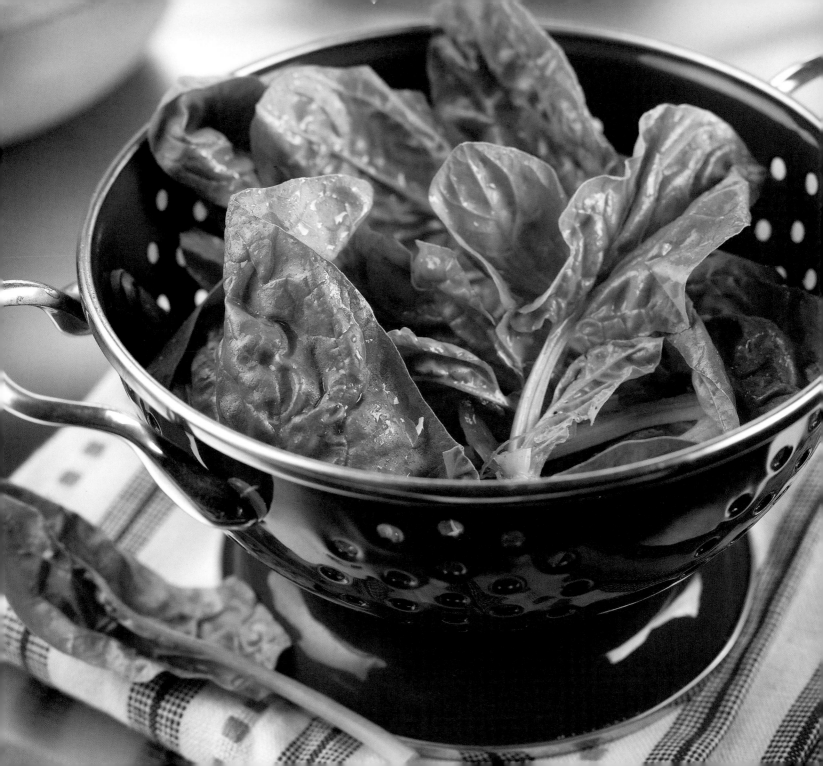

FOOD & FERTILITY

Congratulations! Because you've picked up this book to look inside, you're probably thinking about starting your family, or actively trying, right now. You want to arm yourself with as much information as you can to be healthy and ready for conception. And you want to know more about how the foods you eat can have a direct and indirect effect on your chances of getting pregnant.

It's not a big leap for most of us to imagine that there are links between what we eat and how our bodies, with their myriad of intricate internal systems, perform. As children, we were taught that vegetables would make us grow strong and healthy, and that carrots were good for our eyes, fish was good for our brains, and milk was good for our bones. It made perfect sense to us, even as children, that different parts of the body benefited from the nutrients in different kinds of foods. But until recently, women didn't think of reproductive health as being influenced by diet. The research on how your diet affects your chances of getting pregnant is still in its early stages, but with each when men took the nutrient carnitine, an amino acid derivative. The study found that three months of carnitine treatment produced a significant improvement in sperm movement. Red meat—especially lamb—and dairy products are the primary sources of naturally occurring carnitine. But if a physician recommends this nutrient as a fertility treatment, he's likely to suggest a supplement (called levocarnitine or L-carnitine).

FOLATE

While folate is not directly linked to a woman's chances of getting pregnant, it's vital that women trying to get pregnant consume enough of this B vitamin (also known as B9). Folate (called *folic acid* in vitamins and supplements) is necessary for cell development and growth in pregnancy. Not getting enough of this important vitamin before conception ups the risk of spinal birth defects in a developing baby. Studies have suggested that folic acid may also help reduce the risk of preterm birth, low birth weight, certain other types of birth defects, and recurrent pregnancy loss.

All women of reproductive age should strive to get adequate dietary folate—the form of the vitamin found naturally in foods. The recommended amount is 400 mcg per day for nonpregnant women (pregnant women need more). Good food sources of this nutrient include oranges and citrus fruits, strawberries, whole grains, green leafy vegetables, many beans and legumes, and fortified breads and cereals.

And by the way, it turns out that folic acid is important for men as well. A study at the University of California, Berkeley, School of Public Health looked at the effects of a father's diet on chromosomal abnormalities in sperm and found that men who consumed high levels of folate (more than 700 mcg per day) had up to 30 percent fewer occurrences of a specific chromosomal defect in which the sperm has extra or missing chromosomes. If sperm with these defects fertilize an egg, the result is either miscarriage or children with genetic problems.

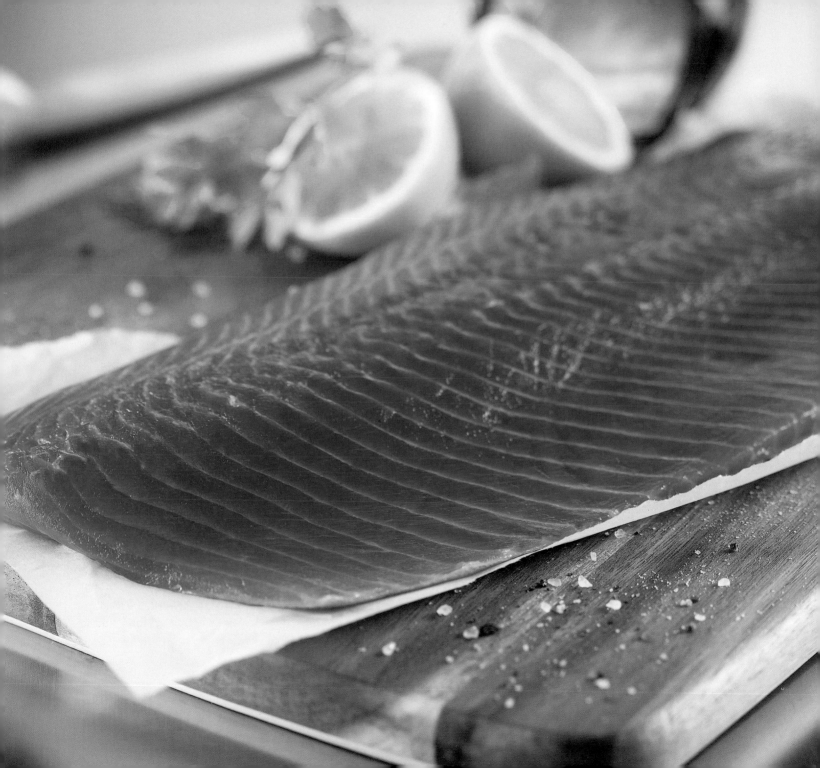

Both you and your spouse can boost the folate in your diet with recipes like Kale and White Bean Ragout with Parmesan Polenta (page 105), Spinach Salad with Grapes and Pecans (page 58), or Wilted Spinach with Garlic (page 155).

FERTILITY FATS

In spite of their bad reputation, not all dietary fats are bad; in fact some are actually beneficial for overall health and, yes, conception. The fat in dairy products may help with ovulation. And other types of fat—such as mono- and polyunsaturated fats—also can help improve your chances of getting pregnant.

WHOLE-MILK DAIRY PRODUCTS

Data collected in the Nurses' Health Study—a comprehensive, long-term look at the diet and lifestyle choices of more than 200,000 female nurses—led to the surprising finding that a daily serving or two of whole milk and foods made from whole milk (full-fat yogurt, cottage cheese, and even ice cream) seem to offer some protection against ovulatory infertility, while skim and low-fat milk do the opposite.

The results, published in 2007, contradict the usual nutritional recommendations to minimize consumption of the kind of saturated fat found in diary products. But the surprising finding does make sense when you consider what's been removed from nonfat and low-fat milk and the foods made from them.

The fat globules in milk contain sex hormones such as estrogen, progesterone, and some androgens (male hormones). When the milk fat is skimmed off, these hormones are removed, too. And researchers think that may be the link between consuming full-fat dairy and ovulation. While the findings don't give you carte blanche to indulge in your favorite pint of ice cream every night, they do mean that if you're thinking about becoming pregnant, you should consider incorporating whole-milk dairy into your diet in nutritious dishes like the Cranberry-Raspberry Smoothie (page 43), Creamy Corn Chowder (page 68), and even Creamy Chocolate Pudding (page 134).

MONO- AND POLYUNSATURATED FATS AND OMEGA-3S

Mono- and polyunsaturated fats reduce inflammation and increase insulin sensitivity, two factors that can disrupt the body's hormone balance. These fats also promote healthy development in a new and rapidly growing embryo.

Avocados, nuts such as cashews and almonds, and seeds such as sesame and pumpkin are all good sources of monounsaturated fats, as are olive oil, canola oil, and peanut oil. Polyunsaturated fats are found in fatty, cold-water fish such as sardines and salmon. These foods contain the type of polyunsaturated fats called *omega-3s*, which are associated with many health benefits and are necessary for a baby's brain development after conception. You'll find several ways to enjoy salmon in this book, including Maple-Glazed Salmon (page 101), and Penne with Salmon, Peas, and Asparagus (page 99). Plant sources of omega-3 fats include flaxseed and walnuts, as well as canola oil, which stars in moist desserts like Pumpkin Gingerbread (page 132).

In general, American diets are too high in omega-6 fatty acids (found in corn and safflower oils), but they tend to neglect the important omega-3s. Too much omega-6 can mediate uterine contractions and lead to early miscarriage even before a woman realizes she's pregnant. That's why it's important for women to learn to balance their intake of these fats and start choosing omega-3s over omega-6s whenever possible . . . even before getting pregnant.

COMPLEX CARBOHYDRATES

These days carbohydrates—or the lack of them—are most often associated with popular weight loss programs. But these dietary elements also have other important functions. Carbohydrates help determine blood sugar and insulin levels. When these

Great Grains

If whole wheat and oats make you yawn, it's time to try some new grains. You can get a little bit adventurous and try brown rice and whole wheat pasta. Or you can really expand your horizons with a world of great grains. Visit your local farmer's market or natural foods store to find kamut, millet, quinoa, amaranth, buckwheat, kasha, and pearl barley. For cooking ideas, ask at the market, search the Web, or just have fun and experiment until you find what tastes good.

levels rise too high, as they do in people with insulin resistance (a breakdown in the body's ability to respond to insulin), they can interfere with the hormone balance necessary for ovulation and reproduction.

Results from the Nurses' Health Study found that it's not the quantity of carbohydrates in a diet that affects fertility, but the type of carbohydrates that are consumed. Specifically, eating a lot of highly refined carbohydrates (such as white bread, potatoes, or sugary sodas) quickly and continually boosts blood sugar and insulin levels and can lower the chances of ovulation and conception. On the other hand, complex carbohydrates—such as whole grains, beans, vegetables, and whole fruits—which don't affect blood sugar and insulin as dramatically, can boost ovulation and conception. We've made choosing the right kind of carbohydrates easier by providing recipes for dishes that incorporate whole-grain breads, whole-wheat flour, stone-ground cornmeal, brown rice, and oatmeal.

ZINC

While zinc plays an important role in normal ovulation and fertilization, it's rare for women to have a zinc deficiency because the mineral is found in all meats, poultry, and milk products. But zinc may be even more important in male fertility, and experts now link zinc levels to semen and testosterone production and overall sperm quality. Men should try to get 11 mg of zinc daily—the amount in a cup of Cheerios or a small T-bone steak, or just two oysters. (Women need roughly 8 mg daily preconception, and 11 mg once they're pregnant.) Other good sources of zinc include mussels, clams, spinach, and pumpkin seeds.

ANTIOXIDANTS

Current darlings of the nutritional research world, antioxidants protect against and repair cellular damage from free radicals (unstable molecules that can bond with and harm normal molecules). A recent study from the Department of Nutritional

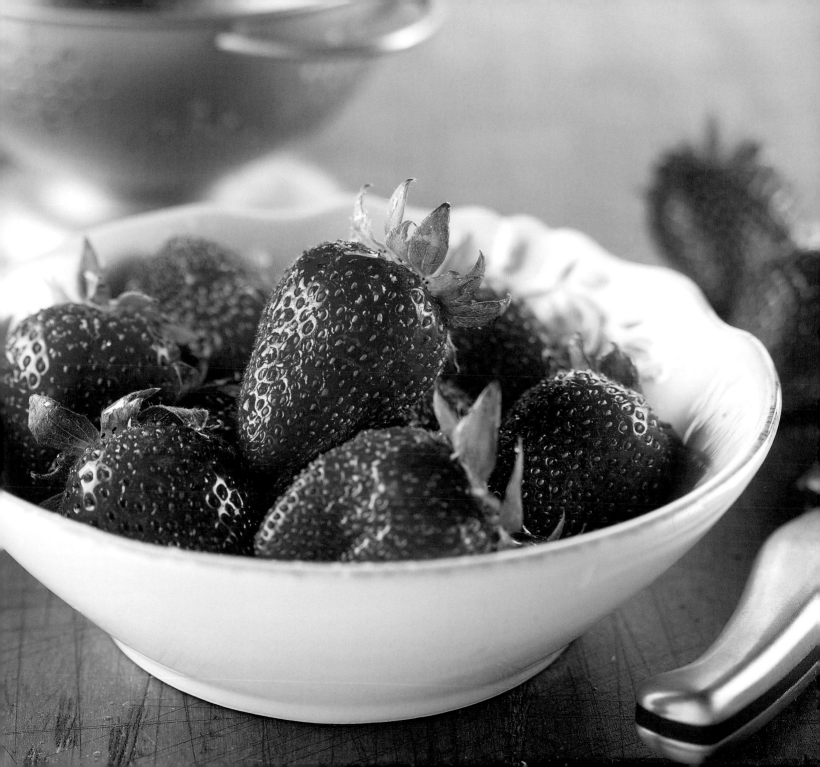

Sciences at Pennsylvania State University suggests that antioxidants' role in preventing and repairing free-radical damage could have implications for female fertility. Other studies have focused on male fertility: Researchers at the University of Rochester found that men who ate the least fresh produce (rich in antioxidants) had the lowest sperm motility. Another study suggested that antioxidant-rich pomegranate juice boosts sperm quality, while yet another found that the antioxidant vitamin C reduces the risk of producing damaged sperm. While studies of antioxidants are still in their infancy, it's clear that these powerful plant compounds, abundant in nuts and colorful fresh fruits and vegetables, have some significant effects on the body's systems. Check out these two male fertility-boosting antioxidants and try to add them to your partner's daily diet:

Lycopene: This antioxidant, responsible for the red coloring in tomatoes, has been found to be lacking in some men with fertility problems. It's thought that lycopene may mop up some of the free radicals that can cause infertility. Researchers at Britain's University of Portsmouth studied the effect of one can of tomato soup a day on healthy men. The results, published in the *British Journal of Urology*, reported that the levels of lycopene in the men's semen rose significantly, and suggested that higher levels of lycopene are associated with increased fertility. The nutrient is more readily absorbed by the body from cooked tomatoes, rather than raw. So try serving your man some Fresh Tomato Soup with Whole-Grain Croutons (page 65) or Linguini with Turkey Bolognese (page 98).

Selenium: The antioxidant mineral *selenium* is also important for male fertility. Scientists at Norwich Laboratory and at the University of Birmingham, both in England, found that fertile males have significantly more selenium in their sperm than infertile men. However, other recent studies have linked excess amounts of

Go Brazilian

All nuts are a source of healthy fat, but one nut also has an exceptionally high amount of the fertility-friendly antioxidant selenium. A man can get the recommended amount (55 micrograms a day) from just a few Brazil nuts. In fact, just 1 ounce of Brazil nuts provides almost 8 times the recommended daily amount. So eat these nuts sparingly.

selenium with decreased sperm quality and increased insulin resistance. Selenium is found in most plant-based foods, but the amount varies depending on the soil in which the plants are grown. The bottom line: get adequate dietary selenium in dishes like Turkey Burgers with Cheddar and Pickled Onions (page 93), but avoid supplements unless your doctor advises otherwise.

PROTEIN

Protein helps to regulate insulin function, and it's important for early fetal development as well. And as with iron, its source seems to make a difference in your chances of becoming pregnant: getting more protein from plants, and less from animals, helps minimize the chances of ovulation problems. In fact, Harvard researchers found that adding just one serving a day of beans, peas, tofu or soybeans, or peanuts or other nuts seemed to help protect against ovulatory infertility. Adding protein from fish or eggs had no effect. But adding one serving a day of red meat, chicken, or turkey was associated with a substantial increase in the risk of ovulation problems. Those findings are a great reason to dine on bean-rich dishes like Kale and White Bean Ragout with Parmesan Polenta (page 105), or Southwest Vegetable Chili (page 106).

THE B VITAMINS

We've already talked about folic acid as an especially important B vitamin, both before and during pregnancy. But other B vitamins play crucial roles, too.

Vitamins B1 (Thiamin) and B3 (Niacin): These Bs aid in glucose metabolism, which is important for insulin function. And what's good for insulin function is good for fertility. Lentils are a great source of both of these vitamins. Corn and black beans are good sources of thiamin; try them in Corn and Black Bean Salsa (page 77).

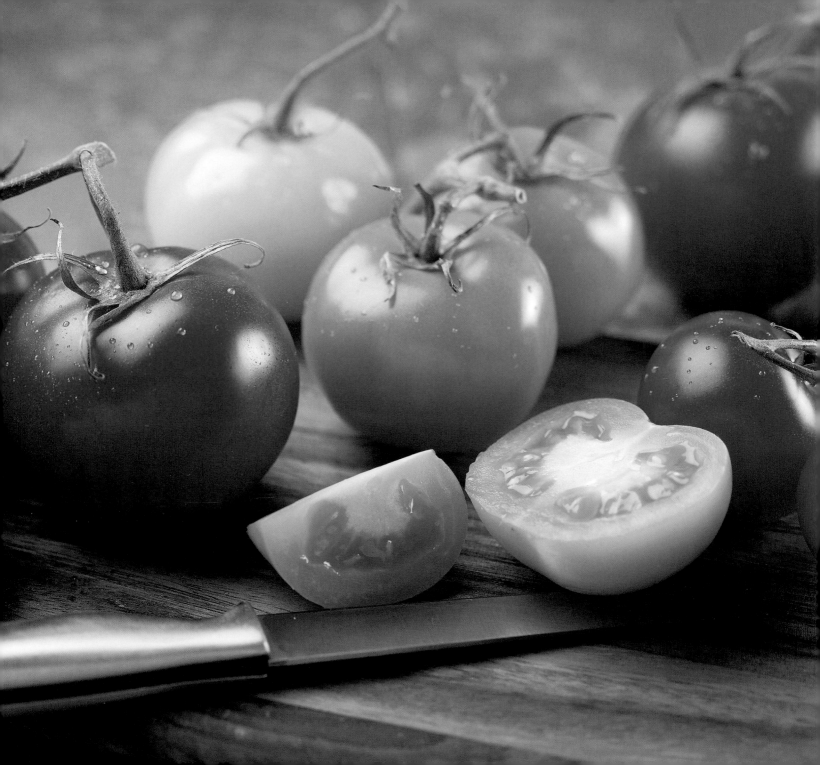

B12: A deficiency in this important vitamin has been linked to miscarriage and to an increased risk of fertility problems. Israeli researchers studying women who'd had repeated miscarriages theorized that B12 deficiencies could cause changes in ovulation or negatively affect the ability of a fertilized egg to implant within the uterus. Meat, fish, milk, and eggs are the primary sources of B12. A dish like Maple-Glazed Salmon (page 101) will give you more than half your RDA. If you're a strict vegetarian, ask your doctor about taking a B12 supplement.

Fertility-Threatening Foods

While we've talked about the foods that may help increase your chances of getting pregnant, other foods have been found to have a negative effect on fertility. Consume the following in moderation, or avoid them entirely for your best chance of conceiving.

TRANS FATS

These artificially manufactured, artery-clogging fats, found in many commercial products and fast foods, should be off your menu entirely, whether you're trying to get pregnant or not. According to the Nurses' Health Study, the more trans fats in a woman's diet, the greater her chance of having fertility problems.

Trans fats are found in stick margarines, vegetable shortening, fast-food french fries and doughnuts, and many packaged foods such as cookies, crackers, and other baked goods. Read labels carefully to avoid these dangerous fats, which have also been linked to heart disease. Look for the words "partially hydrogenated," which means the product contains trans fat.

SOY

The jury is still out on how soy affects male and female fertility. At issue are *isofla-vones*, compounds in soy that behave like estrogen in the body. One study, at King's

College London, found that a compound in soy called *genistein* causes a chemical reaction in sperm as they swim in the female reproductive tract, sabotaging their ability to fertilize the egg. Until more research either confirms or contradicts these findings, it would be smart for men and women hoping to become parents soon to avoid taking supplements of soy protein (read the labels of protein drinks or shakes). And if you regularly consume foods like tofu, soy beans, and soy milk, play it safe and talk to your doctor about whether you should avoid them (at least, for women, around the time of ovulation).

CAFFEINE

Doctors have long warned pregnant women to go easy on caffeine because of its possible role in causing miscarriages. Some studies now suggest that high caffeine intake also may be associated with lessening and delaying a woman's chance of conceiving. But research results have been conflicting, and the effect of caffeine on conception and pregnancy is still not well understood. Most doctors agree that as long as you limit your intake to one or two cups of coffee per day (that's an 8-ounce cup, not a grande size from the neighborhood café) you should be okay. But keep in mind that other foods and drinks contain caffeine, too, including tea, soft drinks, and chocolate. Even some over-the-counter pain relievers contain caffeine. Be aware of the various sources of caffeine in your diet so you can keep your consumption moderate.

ALCOHOL

Many experts say that moderate drinking is okay when you're trying to conceive, although, to be safe, they recommend cutting out alcohol completely as soon as you know you're pregnant. If you're trying to become pregnant and you drink more than occasionally, this is a good time to cut back, or to eliminate alcohol entirely, sooner rather than later. And since many women don't know they're pregnant immediately, the March of Dimes and the Centers for Disease Control and Prevention recommend

No Joe for Joe?

Recommendations to cut down on caffeine while trying to conceive a child hold for men, too. Some research has shown that drinking even average amounts of coffee can increase damage to the DNA in sperm. So to stay on the safe side, fathers-to-be should exercise some caffeine caution and limit their consumption to no more than two cups daily.

that women stop drinking as soon as they start trying to conceive. Men aren't off the hook when it comes to drinking and fertility—excessive alcohol consumption in men can affect testosterone levels and the quality of sperm.

VITAMIN A

In a 2002 paper on nutrition and pregnancy, the American Dietary Association warned against excessive intake of vitamin A, which has been shown to cause birth defects at levels above 10,000 IU daily during early pregnancy. Most multivitamin supplements contain half that amount, but some have as much as 10,000, and supplements aren't the only source of vitamin A. Grains, cereals, and packaged foods like granola bars and cereal bars are sometimes fortified with vitamin A. This doesn't mean you should stop eating carrots, but if you're taking a supplement, check to see how much vitamin A it contains, and keep other sources of vitamin A in your diet at a minimum when you're trying to conceive.

If You're a Vegetarian

If you're a vegetarian, you're in luck! A nutritious vegetarian diet is well suited to support conception and pregnancy. By getting your protein and iron from plant-based sources, you're ahead of the game when it comes to eating for fertility. However, if you're a strict vegetarian or vegan and eat no dairy products or eggs, talk to your doctor about taking a supplement that contains B12, zinc, iron, and calcium while you're trying to conceive.

Vitamins and Supplements

It's good to meet as many of your nutritional requirements as you can from a healthy diet rich in whole foods. That said, even health food fanatics may find it difficult to fit in all the recommended nutrients, which are especially important while you're trying to get pregnant and during pregnancy. Obstetricians recommend special prenatal vitamins during pregnancy, but some doctors are now advising women to start taking these vitamins as soon as they begin trying to conceive. Prenatal vitamins typically have more folic acid, iron, and calcium than regular, one-a-day type vitamins. But even a daily multivitamin is generally sufficient to fill in nutrients that may be missing from your diet and help you prepare your body for pregnancy.

At your preconception checkup (yes, you should have one), ask your doctor's advice on the right vitamin for you, and read the labels carefully because the components of multivitamins and prenatal vitamins, both over-the-counter and prescription, can vary. Do make sure that whichever supplement you take supplies enough of the "big three" prepregnancy and pregnancy nutrients (folic acid, iron, and calcium).

Folic Acid: You need 400 mcg of folic acid per day prepregnancy, and 600 mcg once you're pregnant, to help prevent defects in the neural tube (embryonic spinal cord) and other birth defects. Because it's very difficult to get enough of this critical nutrient from diet alone—even a top source like orange juice has just 74 mcg in a one-cup serving—the Institute of Medicine, which sets the recommended dietary allowance (RDA) for nutrients, recommends that women take a daily pill of either folic acid on its own or in a multivitamin. And since the folate in food is highly sensitive to heat and light, and some of it is destroyed during cooking, you should consider taking a supplement for at least two months before conception. That's the amount of time it takes for the body to build up protective levels of this vitamin.

Iron. Women are advised to get 18 mg of iron per day before pregnancy, and 27 mg per day during pregnancy. It can be difficult to get this much daily iron from the food you eat, and a woman whose body is low in the nutrient before she conceives will have difficulty making up those levels during pregnancy. That's

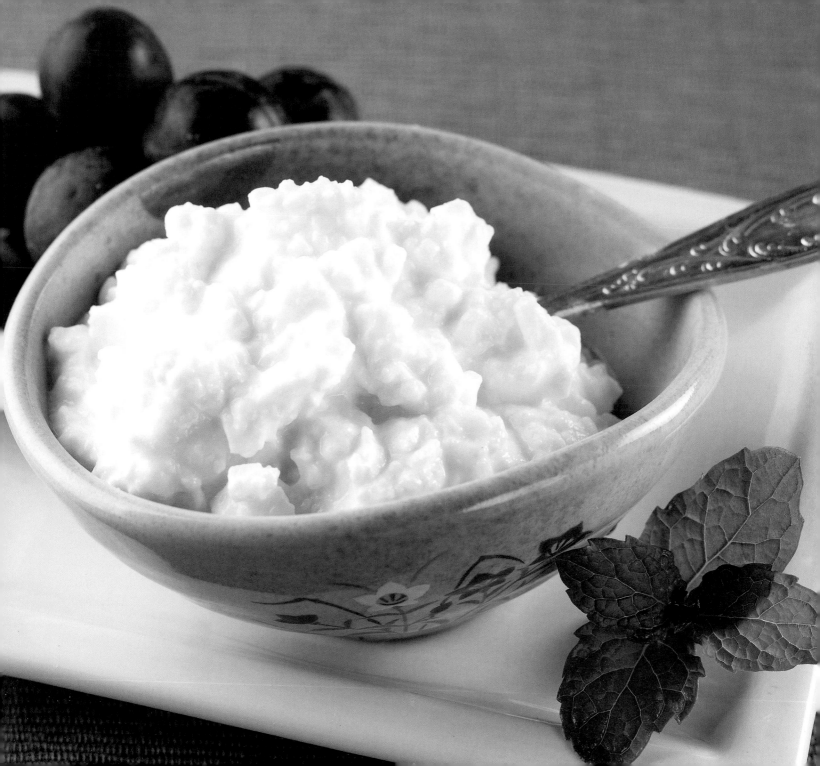

why it's important to build up the body's supply ahead of time, and why you should consider a supplement.

Calcium: Despite years of public health messages, national statistics still show that few women of childbearing age are getting enough calcium. The recommended amount is 1,000 mg per day. And research shows that calcium may be important for more than just mother and baby's bone health. Depressed calcium levels may increase the probability of monozygotic (one-egg) twinning, which can make pregnancies riskier and miscarriage more likely. In research conducted at Long Island Jewish Medical Center, Gary Steinman, M.D., and his colleagues found that thin women with low calcium were especially at risk. Good dietary sources of calcium include milk, cheeses, yogurt, canned salmon, and sardines. Adding a supplement will help you be sure you're getting enough calcium every day.

A Healthy Weight for Conception

Your ideal weight and BMI (body mass index) are dependent upon many factors, including your age, genetics, and your musculature. But there is an optimum weight for becoming pregnant. A BMI of between 20 and 24, (around 21 is ideal), is the range called the "fertility zone."

If you're underweight, with a BMI of under 19, studies suggest that gaining even five pounds can improve your chances of conceiving. When the body's fat stores are low, the hypothalamus, which is the hormone-regulating part of the brain, gets the signal that there's too little body fat and estrogen to support a pregnancy. This can prevent ovulation from occurring. Women who are too thin are also at risk of delivering a low birth weight baby, experiencing a preterm delivery, and becoming anemic during pregnancy. Gaining even a few pounds can help jumpstart ovulation.

On the other hand, too much body fat can cause the body to produce a weaker form of estrogen, which also can prevent ovulation. Plus, being overweight increases risk for pregnancy complications, including high blood pressure and gestational diabetes. If you're overweight, nutritional changes that result in even a modest weight loss can help normalize ovulation and improve your odds of getting pregnant.

A word of caution if you're considering a low-carbohydrate/high-protein approach to weight loss: The effect of a high protein diet on pregnancy has not been studied in humans, but a study involving mice suggested that such a diet could be harmful to the developing embryo. While a nutritionally sound diet during pregnancy is critical, preconception is not the time to try any kind of extreme diet to lose or gain weight. If your BMI is not between 18.5 and 24.9, talk to your doctor about safely losing or gaining a few pounds in preparation for conception.

Men aren't off the hook either when it comes to maintaining a healthy body weight for fertility. While study results have been conflicting, a number of studies have shown that testosterone and sperm production can be adversely affected by being under- or overweight.

PCOS, Weight, Diet, and Fertility

Polycystic ovary syndrome (PCOS) is a leading cause of infertility, and one with a fairly direct link to body weight and dietary changes. In PCOS, the ovaries overproduce male hormones and often produce fluid-filled cysts. The ovaries' functionality, including ovulation, is compromised. Symptoms of PCOS include a long and irregular menstrual cycle, extra hair growth (on the side of the face, the chin, upper lip, nipple area, chest, lower abdomen, thighs), acne, and skin discoloration. Women with PCOS have insulin resistance, which can throw off ovulation, causing subtle changes in the cycle or even making ovulation stop entirely. And one more thing: An estimated 85 to 90 percent of women with PCOS are overweight.

Wake Up & Smell the Cinnamon

No one is claiming that cinnamon rolls are a health food, but studies have shown that cinnamon can improve insulin resistance. Scientists at Columbia University in New York City found that women with PCOS who consumed 1 gram per day of cinnamon extract significantly improved their insulin resistance after eight weeks. So for a possible fertility boost—and a definite taste treat—sprinkle some cinnamon onto your toast, cereal, or yogurt.

Experts aren't sure what causes PCOS. The tendency to develop it may be partly inherited, and lifestyle—specifically a lack of exercise and a diet high in refined carbs—may also play a role. An estimated five to ten million U.S. women suffer from PCOS, but many are undiagnosed and unaware they have the condition.

Here's the good news: PCOS may be a leading cause of infertility, but it's also one that responds well to dietary change and modest weight loss. In one study, 40 percent of obese PCOS patients who lost as little as 5 percent of their body weight (just 10 pounds for a woman who weighs 200 pounds) achieved a spontaneous pregnancy with no other medical treatment. Many doctors now believe that weight loss, dietary change, and exercise are such powerful PCOS treatments that women with the condition who want to conceive should try to make these lifestyle changes for three to six months before they resort to fertility medications or other therapies.

Women with PCOS are not the only ones with insulin resistance; many apparently healthy women may have the condition but are unaware of it. And, just as with PCOS, diet changes and weight loss (if necessary) can help restore fertility. Eating a balanced diet of complex carbohydrates, proteins, and healthy fats can help get the body's insulin levels—and ovulation—back on track. It's estimated that these changes alone could make the difference between conceiving naturally—or not—for up to half of all women who are having difficulty.

Eating Green for Fertility

Much is already known about which nutrients women need and which foods they should eat when trying to get pregnant. But much less is known about how the preservatives, hormones, pesticides, and other toxic chemicals that might be in your food could interfere with your ability to conceive.

Increasing evidence suggests that long-term exposure to the chemicals that are all around us in our everyday environments may play a role in fertility problems ranging from impaired egg production to repeat miscarriage, sperm abnormalities, and decreased sperm counts. As long as you're taking the trouble to choose healthy fertility-supporting foods, there are some important things you should know about keeping that food as free of environmental contaminants as possible.

PITCH THE PLASTIC

Bisphenol-A (BPA) and *phthalates*, both chemicals commonly used in plastics, are big news these days. BPA is a chemical compound in hard plastics like those used for food containers, water bottles, baby bottles, and the lining of many metal food cans. It's been connected (in animal studies) with accelerating puberty and raising the risk of miscarriage as well as having adverse effects on male reproductive development. Phthalates are used to soften plastics (such as shower curtains), as well as to keep the scent or color in health and beauty products and make creams creamier. Even at low levels, phthalates seem to affect estrogen and testosterone. In animal studies, researchers have observed ovulatory irregularities and increased time to achieve pregnancy. When a male fetus is exposed to the chemical, malformations of the reproductive tract and decreased semen quality have been documented. In men, associations have been found between phthalates and decreased sperm motility. Because of these and other concerns, the European Union, Canada, and the United States have already banned some forms of phthalates in certain applications.

To keep these harmful compounds from leaching into your food, store edibles—especially hot food and liquids—in glass, ceramic, or stainless-steel containers instead of plastic. Don't allow plastic cling wrap to come into contact with hot or high-fat foods like cheese. Reduce your use of canned foods in favor of fresh or frozen. Avoid microwaving food in plastic containers, and hand-wash plastic dinnerware and utensils in warm water (not in the dishwasher). Discard any plastic that comes in contact with food if it is scratched or worn. And don't reuse plastic water bottles.

Bottle It Up

You thought you were doing everything right by working out regularly. And you always bring along a handy water bottle to keep yourself healthy and hydrated. But if your water bottle is plastic, you might want to make a switch so you don't get a dose of fertility-threatening chemicals along with your H_2O. Food grade stainless steel water bottles are a good solution, as are new plastic bottles that advertise themselves as BPA- and phthalate-free. Both are readily available from whole foods and camping supply stores.

BUY ORGANIC

According to Robert Greene, M.D., author of *Perfect Hormone Balance for Fertility*, an estimated 90 percent of our total intake of pesticides, fungicides, herbicides, preservatives, additives, and antibiotics comes from the foods we eat. Many of these chemicals are hormone disrupters, which interfere with the body's hormone balance and can reduce fertility or lead to miscarriage. To be on the safe side, some experts advise that if you're thinking about getting pregnant, now is a good time to go organic with at least some of the foods you consume.

If you shop at farmers' markets and local farm stands, you might be surprised to find that organic produce isn't as expensive as it's often reputed to be. But if cost is an issue, spend your organic dollars wisely, on animal products (meat and dairy), and on the fruits and vegetables that would otherwise have the highest pesticide residues. Keep a copy of the list on the opposite page at hand when you shop.

CHOOSE FISH CAREFULLY

Fish is a good source of protein and healthy omega-3 fats, and it's beneficial for pregnancy and conception. But choose your fish wisely to optimize your intake of those healthy omega-3s without exposing yourself to unsafe levels of mercury or other pollutants. Experts generally consider it safest to eat U.S. farmed catfish and wild Alaskan salmon as often as you wish; canned light tuna can be safely eaten up to twice per week. Farmed salmon, shark, swordfish, tilefish, and king mackerel should be avoided. For more information on safe seafood choices, visit the Food and Drug Administration's Web site at www.cfsan.fda.gov/~dms/admehg3.html.

BEST STRATEGY: A HEALTHY, BALANCED DIET

Exposure to toxins is inevitable in this modern world, but there's evidence that the foods you eat can lessen the effects of your exposure. Some studies have shown that it may be possible to block the harmful effects of arsenic, for example, by having a

HIGHEST PESTICIDE RESIDUES	MODERATE PESTICIDE RESIDUES	LOWEST PESTICIDE RESIDUES
Apples	Apricots	Apple juice[†]
Grapes (imported)	Blueberries	Bananas
Nectarines	Cantaloupe	Kiwifruit
Peaches	Grapefruits	Mangoes
Pears	Grapes (domestic)	Orange juice[†]
Red raspberries	Honeydew	Papayas
Strawberries	Oranges	Peaches (canned)
Bell peppers	Collard greens	Pineapples
Carrots	Cucumbers	Plums
Celery	Kale	Tangerines
Green beans	Lettuce	Watermelon
Hot peppers	Mushrooms	Asparagus
Potatoes	Sweet potatoes	Avocados
Spinach	Tomatoes	Broccoli
	Turnip greens	Cabbage
	Winter squash	Cauliflower
		Onions
		Sweet corn
		Sweet peas

List based on analysis of USDA and FDA data (1992–2001) by the Environmental Working Group; items with † based on a study by Consumers' Union of USDA, California Department of Pesticide Regulation, and CU testing data.

Guys, Eat Your Fruits & Veggies

Hey, men, your mom was right about eating fruits and vegetables, especially if she's hoping to be a grandmother. Research at the University of Rochester in New York found that the more fresh produce a man eats, the better his sperm is able to fertilize an egg. Fresh fruits and vegetables are high in antioxidants that protect sperm from damage. Brightly-colored produce such as carrots, tomatoes, blueberries, and oranges are particularly beneficial. So remember the food pyramid, and try to eat at least five servings of fruits and vegetables daily.

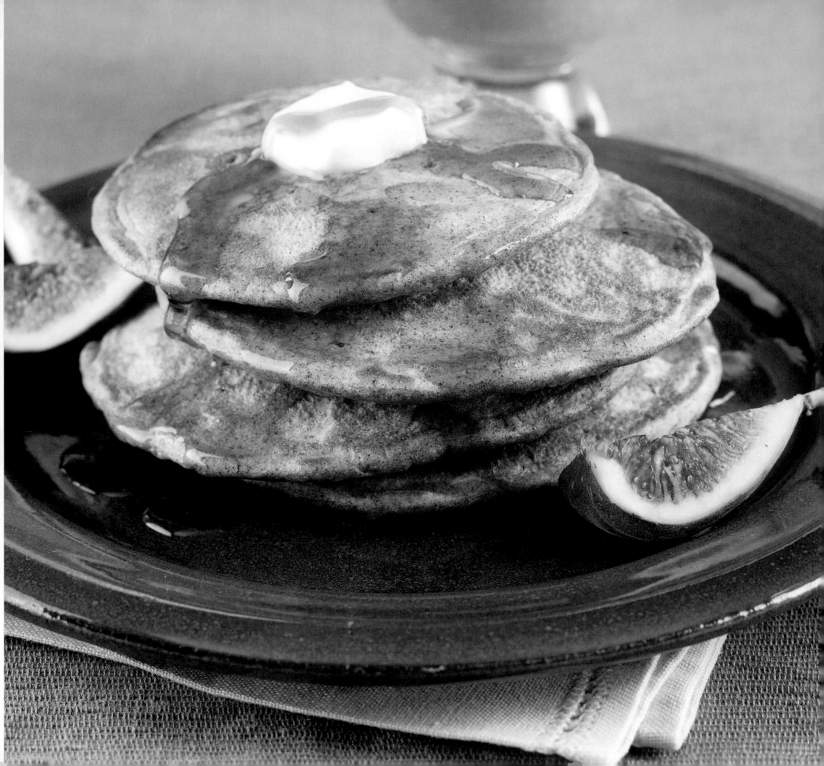

BREAKFAST

You've probably heard plenty about how a healthy breakfast can increase your mental alertness and even make you less likely to over-indulge later in the day. But breakfast is also prime time for getting important fertility-supporting nutrients like calcium, fiber, and protein. In this chapter, you'll find simple, tempting, and nutritious ways to start your day. For weekend mornings or brunch with friends, there are easy make-ahead dishes like the Red and Green Frittata packed with colorful vegetables. You'll find recipes for sweet baked goods like Oatmeal-Raspberry Muffins that you can keep in the freezer for instant weekday breakfasts. There are also plenty of quick fixes in this chapter, including blended smoothies and a variety of savory toppings for bagels, all of which take just minutes to prepare.

Blueberry-Almond Muesli

2 tablespoons (30 ml)
canola oil, plus more for oiling pan

3/4 cup (178 ml)
Grade B maple syrup

1/4 teaspoon (1.25 ml) salt

*2 cups (480 ml) rolled oats**

1 cup (240 ml)
roughly chopped
*raw almonds**

3 tablespoons (45 ml)
*sesame seeds**

1 cup (240 ml)
puffed rice cereal

1/2 cup (120 ml)
unsweetened or
lightly sweetened
bran or corn flakes

1/2 cup (120 ml)
*dried blueberries**

Making your own version of this popular, healthy breakfast cereal ensures that you're getting only the ingredients you need, like fiber and magnesium from the oats, and protein and calcium from the almonds. This mixture of toasted oat clusters, dried blueberries, almonds, and puffed brown rice is delectable topped with fresh fruit and yogurt or milk, which adds more protein and calcium to this breakfast. Choose whole milk or yogurt for the added fertility benefits of whole-milk dairy products.

Serves 10; makes about 5 cups (1.2 liters)

1. Preheat the oven to 325°F (160°C). Lightly oil a large baking pan or jellyroll pan.

2. In a large bowl, whisk together the 2 tablespoons (30 ml) oil, syrup, and salt. Stir in the oats, almonds, and sesame seeds, mixing to coat completely. Spread the mixture in an even layer 1/4-inch (6 mm) thick in the prepared pan and bake, stirring once midway through baking time, until the oats and almonds are golden brown, 25 to 30 minutes. Let cool completely.

3. Stir in the puffed rice, bran flakes, and blueberries and transfer to an airtight container; store at room temperature for up to 2 weeks.

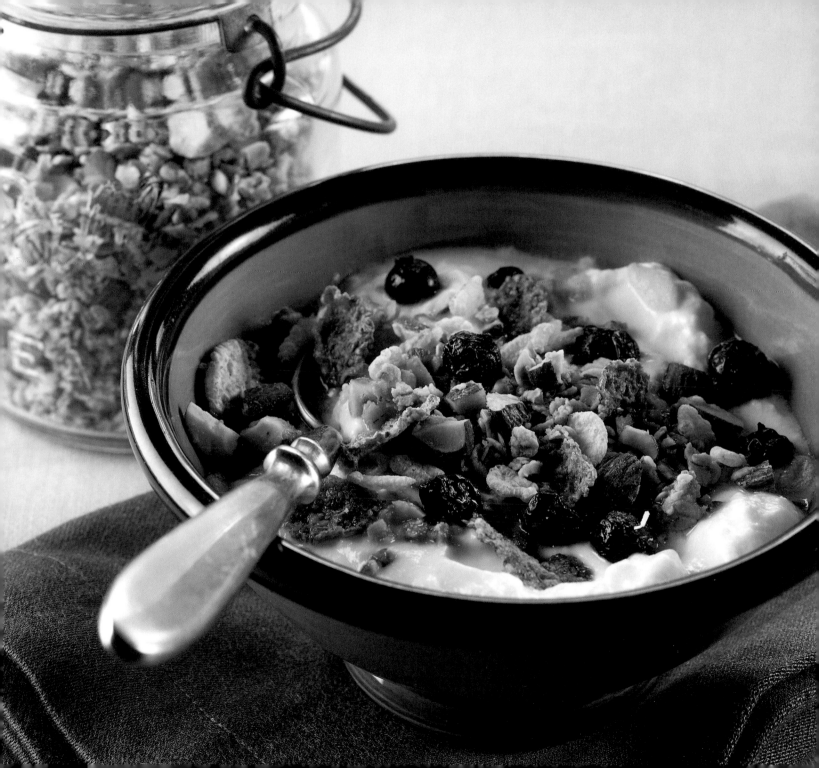

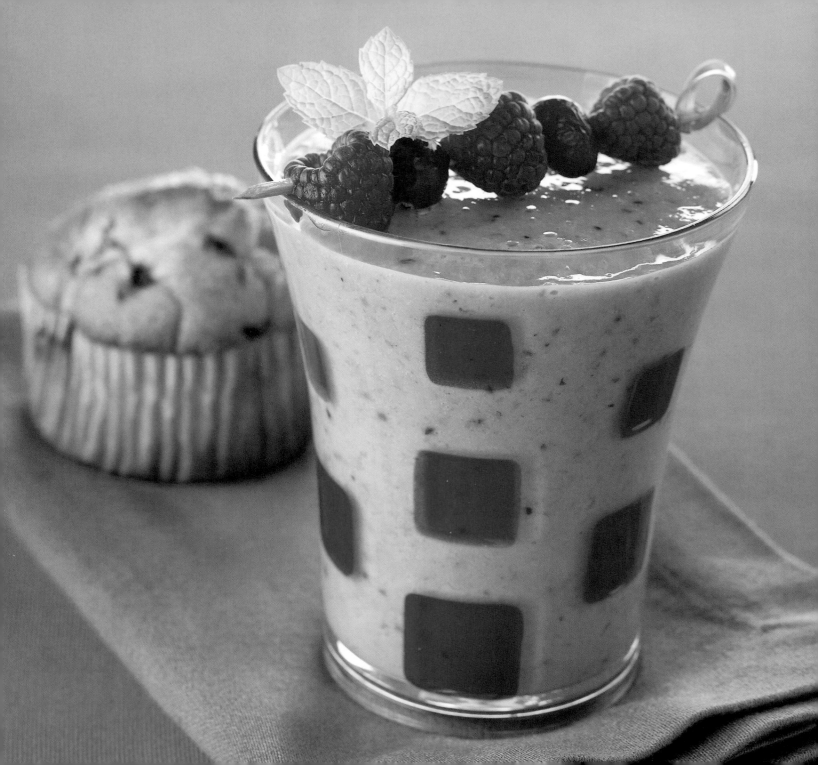

Cranberry-Raspberry Smoothie

A morning smoothie is a great way to get a serving of important fertility foods like calcium-rich yogurt and orange juice, which is a good source of folate. For a thick, icy drink with the texture of a milk shake, freeze a peeled banana the night before you plan to make this smoothie, and use it in the recipe.

Serves 1 to 2; makes 1¹/₂ cups (360 ml)

Combine the banana, raspberries, yogurt, cranberries, orange juice, and 1 tablespoon (15 ml) honey in a blender and whirl until smooth. Taste for sweetness and add more honey, if desired. If you used a frozen banana, you may need to add more orange juice to thin the smoothie to your desired consistency.

1 ripe banana, peeled, fresh or frozen

1/2 cup (120 ml) fresh raspberries*

1/2 cup (120 ml) vanilla or plain whole-milk yogurt*

2 tablespoons (30 ml) fresh or frozen cranberries*

1/2 cup (120 ml) fresh orange juice*

1 to 2 tablespoons (15 to 30 ml) honey

FERTILITY FACT:

Getting enough folic acid before pregnancy is important to help prevent serious spinal birth defects. Citrus fruits and orange juice are a great source of this B vitamin.

Red and Green Frittata

6 cups (1.4 liters)
bite-size broccoli florets*

8 large eggs*

¼ cup (60 ml) milk

¼ teaspoon (1.25 ml) salt

¼ teaspoon (1.25 ml)
freshly ground pepper

1 red bell pepper, cut into
¼-inch (6 mm) thick slices*

1 cup (4 ounces or 113 grams)
grated white Cheddar or
fontina cheese, divided*

4 tablespoons (60 ml)
grated Parmesan
cheese, divided

2 teaspoons (10 ml) olive oil

Eggs contain protein and iron, important nutrients for fertility. Broccoli is a good source of folate and fiber. This baked frittata, full of colorful vegetables, is a delicious way to eat them, for brunch or a light lunch or supper.

Serves 6 to 8

1. Bring a large pot of water to a boil; add the broccoli and cook until just tender, about 3 minutes. Drain well.

2. Preheat the oven to 350°F (180°C). In a large bowl, whisk the eggs, milk, salt, and pepper together in a large bowl. Stir in the broccoli, red pepper, ¾-cup (36 ounces) of the Cheddar, and 3 tablespoons (45 ml) of the Parmesan cheese.

3. Heat the oil in a 12-inch (305 mm) ovenproof nonstick frying pan over medium-high heat. Pour the egg mixture into the pan and reduce the heat to medium. Cook for 3 minutes to set the bottom of the frittata. Sprinkle the top with the remaining ¼-cup of the Cheddar (12 ounces) and 1 tablespoon (15 ml) Parmesan cheese.

4. Transfer the pan to the oven and bake until the frittata is set in the center and slightly puffy, about 15 minutes.

5. Let cool for 5 minutes in the pan, and then run a spatula around the edges and slide onto a large plate. Cut into wedges and serve.

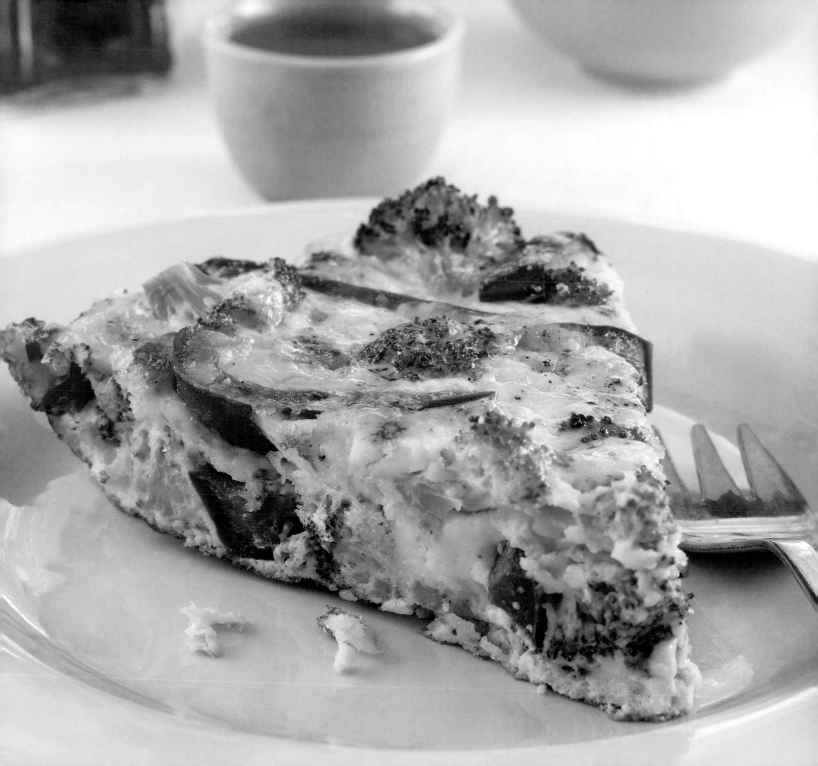

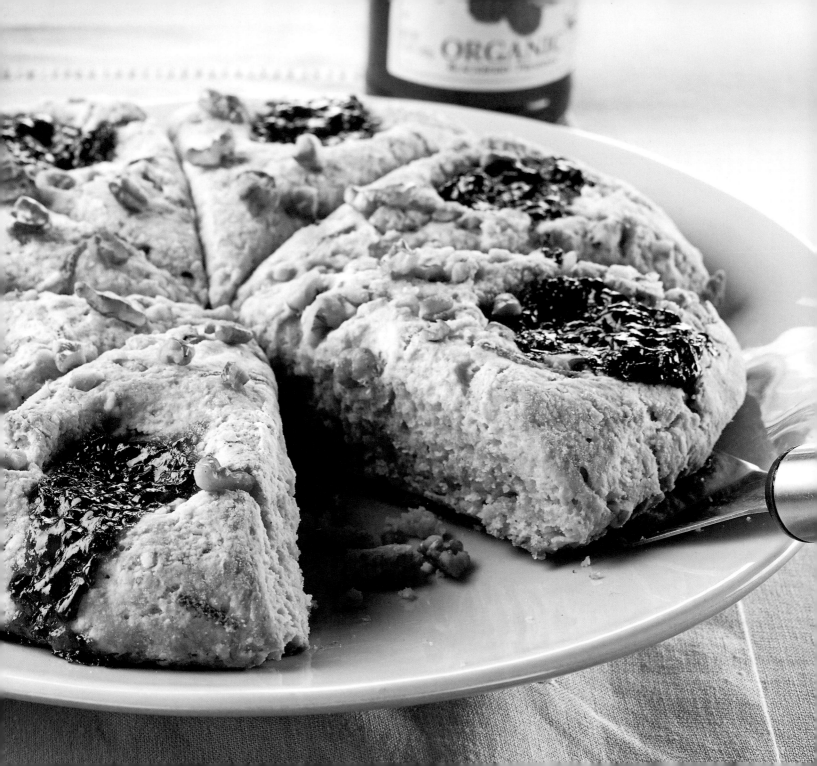

Walnut Scones with Blackberry Jam Thumbprints

Walnuts are packed with important omega-3s. Whole-wheat flour gives the scones extra fiber. These crumbly, delicious whole-wheat-and-walnut scones have a spoonful of jam baked into them. Use fruit preserves made without added sugar, or use organic preserves if you prefer. You can bake these on the weekend, freeze them, and then defrost them for easy week-day breakfasts.

Makes 8 scones

1. Preheat the oven to 375°F (190°C). Butter a large baking sheet, or line it with a sheet of cooking parchment.

2. In a bowl, mix the flours, sugar, baking powder, and salt. Add the butter and use a fork or your fingertips to rub the butter into the dry ingredients until the mixture resembles coarse crumbs.

3. In a small bowl, whisk together the buttermilk, egg, and vanilla. Add to the flour mixture along with the 1/2 cup (120 ml) walnuts and the orange zest. Stir with a fork until the dough is evenly moistened and starts to come together into a ball (dough will look crumbly; add another tablespoon of buttermilk if the dough is too dry to come together).

4. Scrape the dough onto a lightly floured board and knead a few times. Pat the dough into a 10- to 12-inch (25- to 30-cm) round. Slide the round onto the prepared baking sheet and cut into 8 wedges, leaving the wedges in place. Use your thumb to make a depression 1 inch (2.5 cm) in diameter on the wide end of each wedge and use a spoon to fill each with about 1/2 tablespoon (1.5 ml) jam. Sprinkle tops of scones with remaining 2 tablespoons (30 ml) chopped walnuts.

5. Bake until golden brown, 25 to 28 minutes. Recut scones to separate, and serve warm, or transfer to a rack to cool completely.

1 cup (240 ml)
all-purpose flour

2 cups (480 ml)
whole-wheat flour*

1/4 cup (60 ml) sugar

1 tablespoon (15 ml)
baking powder

1/2 teaspoon (2.5 ml) salt

6 tablespoons (90 ml)
cold butter, cut into chunks

1 cup (240 ml) buttermilk
(low fat or regular)*

1 large egg*

2 teaspoons (10 ml)
vanilla extract

1/2 cup (120 ml) plus
2 tablespoons (30 ml)
finely chopped walnuts*

2 teaspoons (10 ml)
grated orange zest

1/4 cup (60 ml)
blackberry preserves

Fluffy Buckwheat Pancakes

1 cup (240 ml)
all-purpose flour

1 cup (240 ml)
buckwheat flour*

1 teaspoon (5 ml)
baking powder

1/2 teaspoon (2.5 ml)
baking soda

1/4 teaspoon (1.25 ml) salt

3 large eggs,
separated*

1 3/4 cups (418ml)
buttermilk*

1 tablespoon (15 ml)
canola oil, plus
more for oiling pan

1/8 teaspoon (.5 ml)
cream of tartar

Maple syrup for serving

Nutty buckwheat flour has been associated with reduced insulin resistance and increased ovulation in women with PCOS (polycystic ovary syndrome). Serve these pancakes with fresh figs or strawberries and real maple syrup, or fruit preserves made without added sugar. This recipe doubles easily to serve a crowd.

Serves 3 to 4; makes 10 to 12 pancakes

1. In a large bowl, stir together the flours, baking powder, baking soda, and salt. In a small bowl, beat the egg yolks, buttermilk, and the 1 tablespoon (15 ml) oil until well blended. Stir the buttermilk mixture into the flour mixture just until evenly moistened.

2. In a bowl using a mixer on high speed, whip the egg whites with cream of tartar until soft peaks form. Fold gently into the batter until no white streaks remain.

3. Heat a 12-inch (30 mm) nonstick frying pan or a nonstick griddle over medium heat. Coat the pan lightly with about 1/2 teaspoon (2.5 ml) oil and carefully wipe off excess with a paper towel. Working in batches, spoon batter into the pan in 1/3-cup (80 ml) portions and cook until the pancakes are browned on the bottom and a few bubbles have popped on the surface, about 2 minutes. Flip the pancakes and cook the other side until the underside is well browned and the pancakes are cooked through, about 2 minutes longer. Repeat to make the remaining pancakes, adding more oil to the pan as necessary.

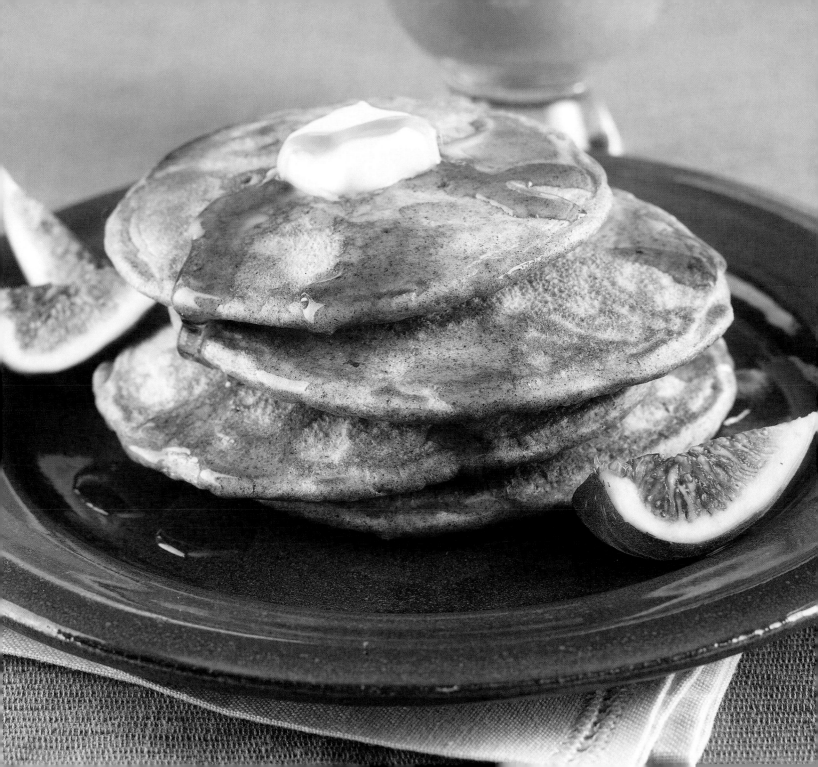

Spinach and Mushroom Omelet with Ricotta Cheese

3 large eggs*

2 tablespoons (30 ml) milk (whole or 1 or 2 percent)*

Salt

Pepper

4 teaspoons (20 ml) olive oil, divided

1/3 cup (80 ml) sliced brown or button mushrooms (about 1 ounce or 28 grams)*

1/8 teaspoon (.5 ml) dried thyme

1/3 cup (80 ml) baby spinach leaves, washed *

1/3 cup (80 ml) whole-milk ricotta cheese*

Leafy spinach is full of calcium, iron, folate, and magnesium, making it a great omelet filling if you're trying to get pregnant! If you've never cooked an omelet before, you'll be surprised how easy it is. If you want to make two, you can double the filling ingredients and cook them together, but cook the omelets one at a time.

Serves 1 to 2

1. Crack the eggs into a bowl. Add the milk and 1/4 teaspoon (1 ml) each of salt and pepper. Beat with a fork until well blended; set aside.

2. Heat 2 teaspoons (10 ml) of the oil in a nonstick frying pan over medium-high heat. Add the mushrooms and sprinkle lightly with salt and pepper. Add the thyme and stir until the mushrooms are browned, 4 to 6 minutes. Add the spinach and stir until wilted, 1 to 2 minutes. Transfer the mushroom mixture to a bowl and set aside.

3. Heat the remaining oil in the frying pan and then slowly pour in the egg mixture, tilting the pan to cover the bottom of the pan evenly. Let the eggs cook for about 15 seconds. As the egg mixture begins to set, lift the edge with a spatula and tilt the pan slightly to let uncooked egg flow underneath. Repeat this around the sides of the pan until the surface is moist but nearly set. Spoon the ricotta and the mushroom mixture over half of the omelet. With the spatula, fold the omelet in half over the filling.

4. Slide the omelet onto a plate and serve immediately.

Mocha-Banana Smoothie

When you've just got to have it, a little decaffeinated espresso goes a long way in this frosty breakfast drink. A ripe banana provides the sweetness, but if you like it sweeter, add a little honey to taste. For a thick, icy drink with the texture of a milk shake, freeze a peeled banana the night before you plan to make this smoothie and use it in the recipe.

Serves 1 to 2; makes 1½ cups (360 ml)

Combine all of the ingredients in a blender and whirl until smooth. If you used a frozen banana, you may need to add more milk to thin the smoothie to your desired consistency.

*1 ripe banana, peeled, fresh or frozen**

1 teaspoon (5 ml) instant decaffeinated espresso powder

*3/4 cup (178 ml) milk**

1 tablespoon (15 ml) cocoa powder

FERTILITY FACT:
A little bit of coffee is fine when you're trying to conceive, but don't overdo it. Most experts recommend keeping caffeine intake to no more than 300 mg daily while trying to conceive (an 8-ounce cup of coffee can have 65 to 120 mg).

Avocado, Grapefruit, and Sunflower Seed Salad

1 ruby grapefruit*

1 large, firm, ripe avocado*

1 head butter lettuce (about
6 to 8 ounces or 168 to 224 grams),
leaves separated, rinsed, crisped,
and torn into bite-size pieces*

¼ cup (60 ml) hulled
sunflower seeds*

3 tablespoons (45 ml)
olive oil

2 tablespoons (30 ml)
rice vinegar

1 tablespoon (15 ml)
fresh lime juice

Salt

Freshly ground pepper

Avocados are a good source or monounsaturated fat and folate, grapefruit contains lycopene, and sunflower seeds are full of iron and omega-3s. They all go together deliciously in this pretty salad, which goes well with Grilled Chicken Fajitas (page 92) or Pumpkin Macaroni and Cheese (page 96).

Serves 4

1. With a sharp knife, cut the peel and outer membrane from the grapefruit. To release the fruit segments, hold the grapefruit over a large bowl and cut between the membrane and fruit. Reserve the fruit and juices; discard the peel and membrane.

2. Cut the avocado in half, pry out and discard the pit, then pull the skin from the avocado and discard. Slice thinly and add to the grapefruit along with the lettuce and the sunflower seeds.

3. In a small bowl, whisk together the oil, vinegar, and lime juice until blended; season to taste with salt and pepper.

4. Pour the dressing over the lettuce mixture and toss gently to coat. Serve immediately.

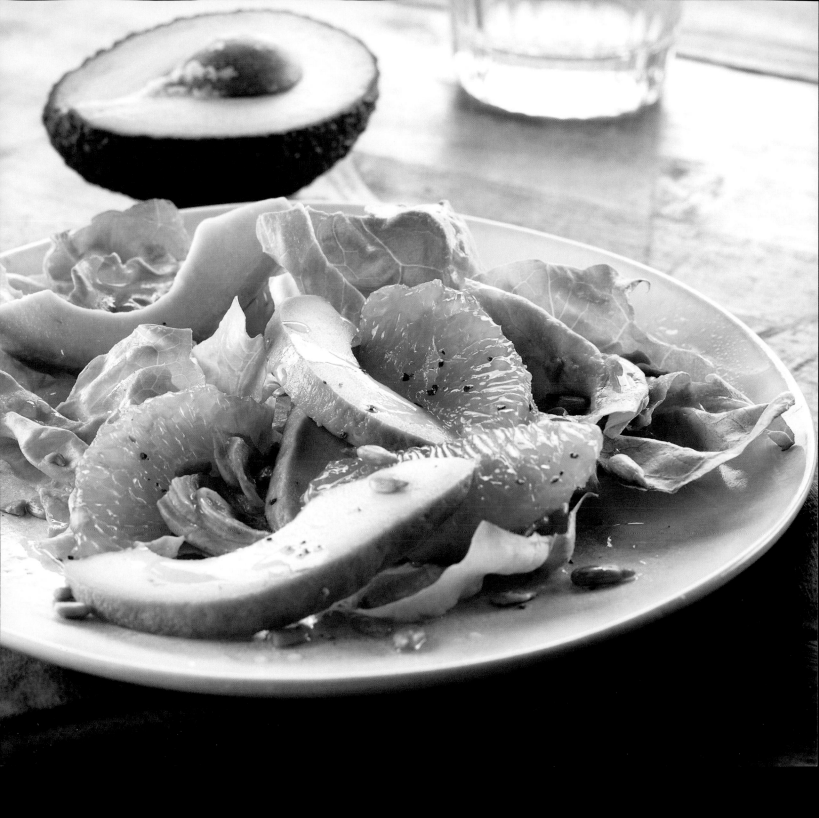

Spinach Salad with Grapes and Pecans

*8 ounces (227 grams)
baby spinach leaves, washed**

*1 cup (240 ml) seedless red flame
grapes, rinsed and halved**

*1/2 cup (120 ml) chopped
pecans, toasted**

*1/2 cup (120 ml) plain
whole-milk yogurt**

*2 tablespoons (30 ml)
cider vinegar*

1 tablespoon (15 ml) honey

*1 tablespoon (15 ml)
poppy seeds*

*1/2 teaspoon (2.5 ml)
grated orange zest*

1/4 teaspoon (1 ml) salt

Spinach salads like this one are a great way to get important iron, calcium, and magnesium. Pecans are a good source of omega-3s and add a nice crunch. To toast the pecans, place them on a baking sheet in a 350°F (180°C) oven until golden and fragrant, 6 to 8 minutes.

Serves 4

Place the spinach, grapes, and pecans in a large bowl. In a small bowl, stir together the yogurt, vinegar, honey, poppy seeds, orange zest, and salt until well blended. Divide the spinach mixture evenly among 4 plates, and drizzle the dressing over each serving. Serve immediately.

Chopped Salad with Turkey and Vegetables

This vegetable-packed Cobb salad is a good way to use leftover roasted turkey breast and get a boost of fiber, folate, and iron, among other important nutrients.

Serves 4

1. Cook the bacon in a frying pan over medium heat until crisp. Place on a paper towel to drain.

2. In a large bowl, mix the vinegar, oil, and mustard until well blended. Add the lettuce and toss well.

3. Mound the lettuce on a large platter. Arrange the remaining ingredients, including the bacon, over the lettuce. Sprinkle lightly with salt and pepper.

4 slices turkey bacon, diced

2 tablespoons (30 ml) red wine vinegar

2 tablespoons (30 ml) olive oil

1 teaspoon (5 ml) Dijon mustard

1 small head red or green leaf lettuce, shredded*

2 cups (480 ml) cubed roasted or cooked turkey breast*

1 cup (240 ml) cherry tomatoes, stemmed and halved*

1 ripe avocado, peeled, pitted, and cubed*

6 ounces (170 grams) Cheddar cheese, cubed*

1 can (15 ounces or 425 grams) chickpeas (garbanzo beans), rinsed and drained*

6 to 8 radishes, stemmed and cut into thin slices*

Salt

Pepper

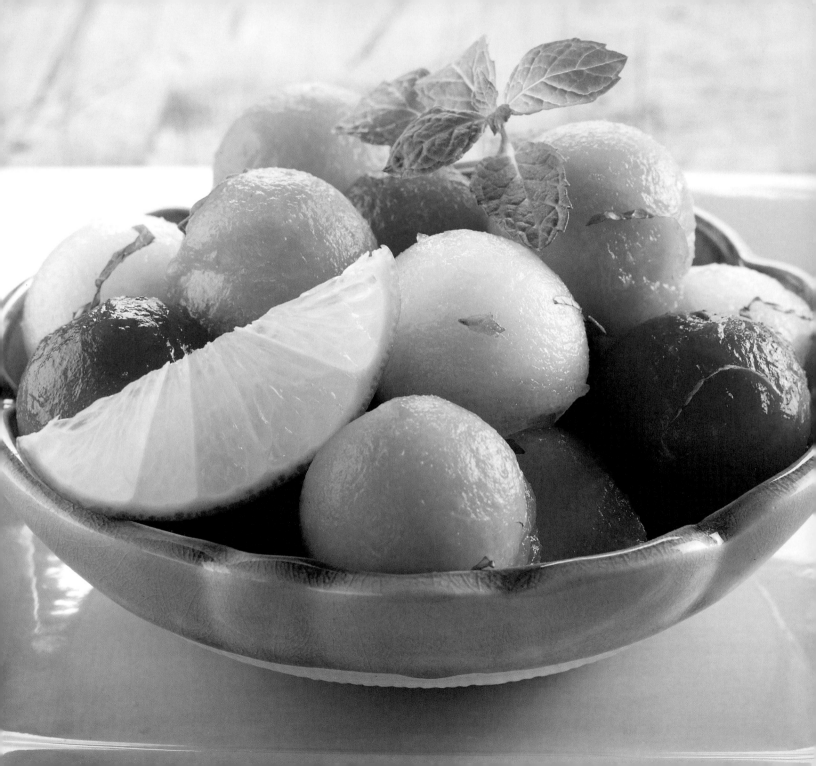

Marinated Melon Salad

This pretty, low-calorie summer salad uses three different colors of ripe, fragrant melon, which is high in potassium, fiber, and vitamins A and C. Watermelon is high in antioxidants, including lycopene. Use a melon baller, if you have one, or just cut the melon into 1-inch (2.5 cm) chunks.

Serves 4

1. In a large bowl, combine the orange juice, lime juice, and salt.

2. Gently stir in the melon. Cut the mint leaves lengthwise into thin strips. Add to the bowl and mix gently. Cover and chill for at least 30 minutes or up to 4 hours. Mix gently before serving.

*3 tablespoons (45 ml) fresh orange juice**

3 tablespoons (45 ml) fresh lime juice

1/4 teaspoon (1.25 ml) salt

*1 cup (240 ml) seedless watermelon, cut into balls or 1-inch (2.5 cm) chunks**

*1 cup (240 ml) honeydew, cut into balls or 1-inch (2.5 cm) chunks**

*1 cup (240 ml) cantaloupe, cut into balls or 1-inch (2.5 cm) chunks**

2 tablespoons (30 ml) lightly packed fresh mint leaves

FERTILITY FACT:
The more fresh fruits and vegetables a man eats, the better his sperm is able to fertilize an egg. Fresh produce contains antioxidants that help protect sperm from damage.

Tabbouleh Salad with Tomatoes and Herbs

1 cup (240 ml) bulgur*

3 tablespoons (45 ml) extra-virgin olive oil*

2 tablespoons (30 ml) balsamic or red wine vinegar

1 tablespoon (15 ml) fresh lemon juice

1/4 teaspoon (1 ml) salt

Freshly ground pepper

1 1/2 cups (356 ml) chopped ripe red and yellow tomatoes*

1 cup (240 ml) canned chickpeas (garbanzo beans), rinsed and drained*

1/4 cup (60 ml) chopped and seeded cucumber

2 tablespoons (30 ml) packed fresh cilantro leaves

1/2 cup (120 ml) chopped fresh parsley leaves

1/4 cup (60 ml) minced red onion

This tangy, fiber-rich salad is a great meatless main dish option. Tomatoes are a good source of vitamin C and lycopene. Feel free to substitute whatever fresh herbs you have on hand.

Serves 4

1. Place the bulgur in a bowl. Pour 3/4 cup (178 ml) boiling water over the bulgur. Cover the bowl and let stand for 30 minutes.

2. In a bowl, combine the oil, vinegar, lemon juice, salt, and pepper. Drain any remaining water from the bulgur and add it to the oil mixture along with the remaining ingredients. Mix the salad gently and season to taste with additional salt and pepper if desired. Serve immediately, or cover and refrigerate for up to 1 day.

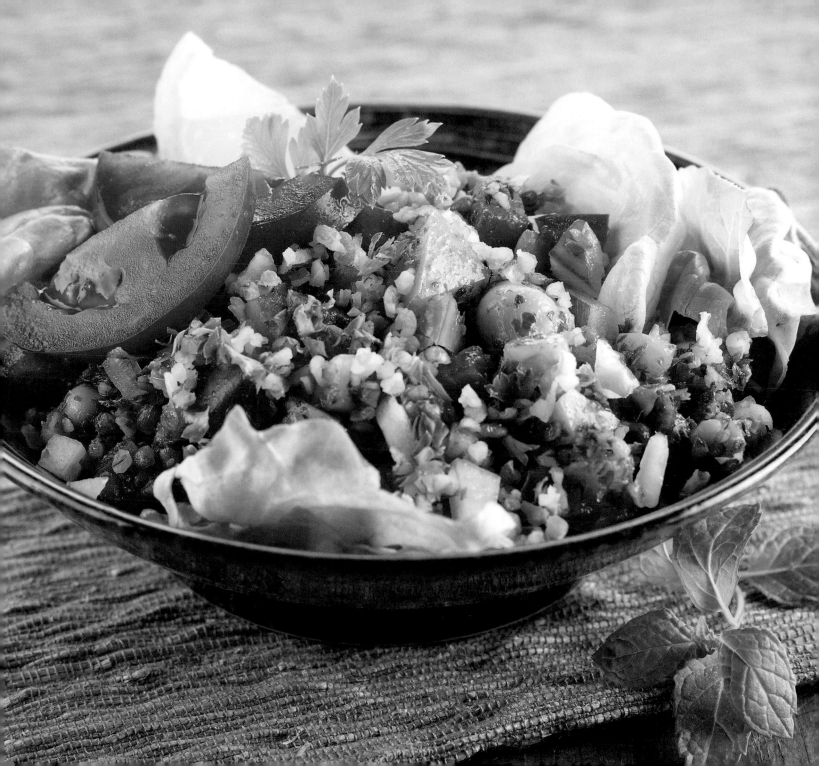

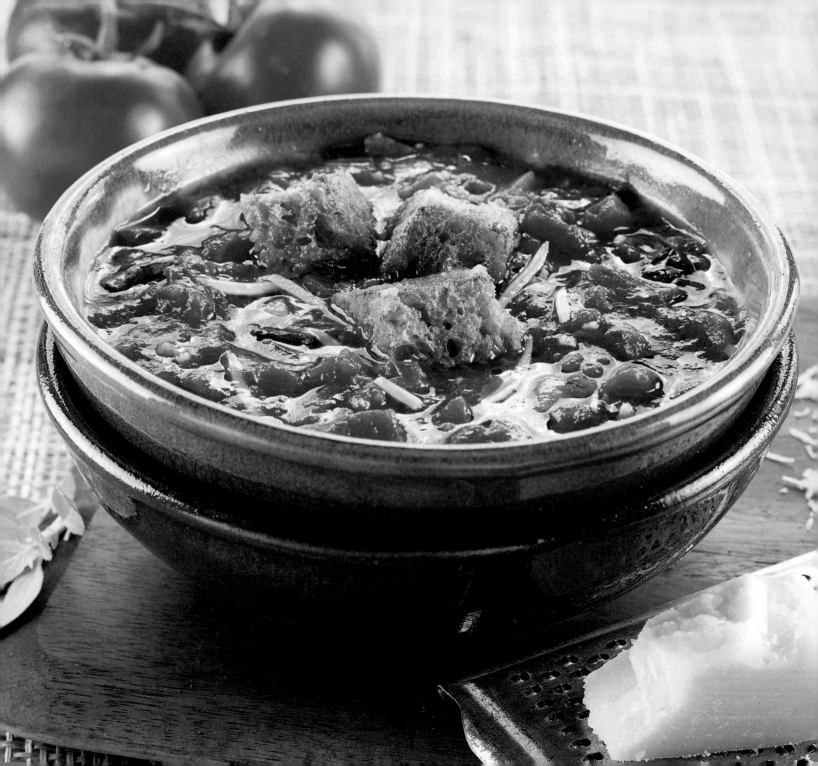

Fresh Tomato Soup with Whole-Grain Croutons

Tomatoes are a good source of lycopene, which is important for sperm production. This simple, low-cal soup is a great way to enjoy them. The whole-grain croutons dissolve into the chunky, rich soup, giving it an earthy texture.

Serves 4

1. Core tomatoes and cut in half crosswise. Gently squeeze over a large bowl to catch juices. Coarsely chop tomatoes and add to bowl.

2. Heat the oil in a large pot over medium heat. Add the garlic and cook just until fragrant, about 45 seconds. Add the tomatoes and the broth. Bring to a simmer, reduce heat and cook 10 to 15 minutes to blend flavors.

3. Stir in basil and season with salt and pepper. Spoon into bowls and top each with croutons and about 1 tablespoon (15 ml) Parmesan cheese.

*3 1/2 pounds (1.6 kilograms) tomatoes**

2 tablespoons (30 ml) olive oil

1 clove garlic, thinly sliced

2 cups (473 ml) chicken broth

1/3 cup (80 ml) packed fresh basil leaves

Salt

Freshly ground pepper

3 slices crusty whole-grain bread, toasted and torn into rough chunks

1/4 cup (60 ml) shredded Parmesan cheese for garnishing

Vegetable Minestrone

2 tablespoons (30 ml) olive oil

1 onion, peeled and chopped

1 carrot, peeled and diced*

1 clove garlic, minced

1 zucchini, diced*

3 cups (720 ml)
chicken broth or water

1 can (28 ounces or 800 grams)
diced tomatoes*

1/4 teaspoon (1.25 ml)
dried oregano

1/4 teaspoon (1.25 ml) salt

Freshly ground pepper

1/3 cup (80 ml) dried orzo
or tiny macaroni

1 can (14.5 ounces or 425 grams)
white beans, drained*

1/4 cup (60 ml) shredded
Parmesan cheese

This simple vegetarian soup comes together quickly, and it's packed with beans, which are a good source of fiber and nonheme iron. If you'd like, turn a crusty whole-grain loaf into garlic bread to accompany the soup.

Serves 4

1. Heat the oil in a large pot over medium-high heat. Add the onion, carrot, and garlic. Stir frequently, reducing the heat as necessary to prevent scorching, until the vegetables soften, about 5 minutes. Add the zucchini, broth, tomatoes, oregano, salt, and a few grinds of pepper. Bring to a boil. Reduce the heat to maintain a simmer. Cover and cook until the vegetables are tender, 15 to 20 minutes.

2. Meanwhile, bring a small pot of water to a boil. Add the pasta and cook until al dente, 8 to 10 minutes. Drain and set aside.

3. Stir the beans into the soup and cook for 5 minutes more to blend the flavors. Then stir in the pasta and Parmesan cheese and serve.

Lentil Soup with Tomatoes, Sausage, and Pesto

A spoonful of pesto garnishes this satisfying fall soup, which is full of iron, protein, folate, and fiber. If you have a bit of Parmesan cheese rind, throw it in the pot while it's simmering to flavor the broth. Look for firm sausage in the refrigerated section of the grocery store, labeled "fully cooked" or "cured."

Serves 4 to 6

1. Heat the oil in a large pot over medium heat. When hot, add the sausage and cook, stirring frequently, until browned, about 5 minutes. Transfer to a plate and set aside. Add the onion, garlic, carrot, and celery to the pot and cook, stirring frequently, until the vegetables are soft, about 5 minutes.

2. Stir in the broth, lentils, tomatoes, cumin, paprika, salt, and pepper. Bring to a boil. Reduce the heat to maintain a simmer, cover, and cook until the lentils are very tender, about 25 minutes. Stir in the sausage and cook until heated through. Ladle into bowls and garnish each serving with a spoonful of the pesto and a sprinkling of the Parmesan cheese.

---

1 tablespoon (15 ml) olive oil

6 ounces (170 grams) cooked turkey or chicken sausage, cut into 1/4-inch (6.4 mm) rounds

1 yellow onion, chopped

1 clove garlic, minced

1 carrot, peeled and diced*

1 stalk celery, diced

4 cups (.95 liter) chicken broth or water

1 cup (240 ml) dried brown lentils, rinsed*

1 can (28 ounces or 800 grams) diced tomatoes*

1 teaspoon (5 ml) ground cumin

1/2 teaspoon (2.5 ml) paprika

1/2 teaspoon (2.5 ml) salt

1/4 teaspoon (1.25 ml) pepper

1/4 cup (60 ml) purchased pesto sauce*

1/4 cup (60 ml) grated Parmesan cheese

Creamy Corn Chowder

5 to 6 ears corn (about 5 cups or 1.2 liters of kernels)*

1 tablespoon (15 ml) olive oil

1 small red onion, chopped

2 teaspoons (10 ml) minced serrano or jalapeño chile

3 cups (720 ml) milk*

1/2 cup (120 ml) vegetable broth, chicken broth, or water (optional)

6 to 8 large fresh basil leaves

1 teaspoon (5 ml) grated lime zest

Sea salt

Freshly ground pepper

Fresh lime juice

This fresh, simple soup is a summertime comfort food, and a great way to get the fertility-enhancing benefits of whole-milk dairy products. Pair it with a salad or a sandwich for lunch or dinner.

Serves 4

1. Husk the corn and, using a small sharp knife and holding the ears over a deep bowl, slice the kernels off the cobs.

2. Heat the olive oil in a medium pot over medium heat. Add the onion; cook and stir frequently until soft, about 5 minutes. Stir in the corn kernels and chile and cook for 2 minutes more.

3. Add the milk and bring to a simmer. Reduce the heat to maintain a gentle simmer, cover, and cook for 15 minutes.

4. With a strainer or a slotted spoon, remove about 2 cups (480 ml) of cooked corn kernels from the soup and set aside. Whirl the remaining soup, in batches if necessary, in a blender or food processor until smooth (taking care because hot liquids may splatter). Return the soup to the pot and stir in the reserved whole corn kernels. Add broth or liquid (if desired) to thin the soup to desired consistency. Roughly tear the basil leaves and stir into the soup. Reheat gently and stir in the lime zest. Season to taste with salt, pepper, and lime juice.

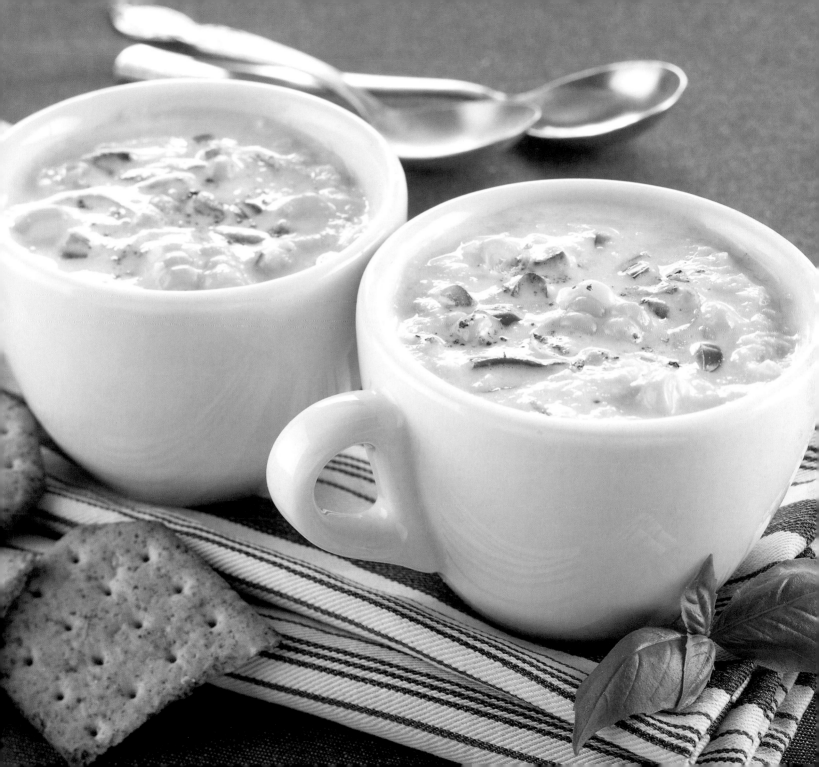

Butternut Squash–Apple Soup

2 tablespoons (30 ml) olive oil

1 yellow onion, finely chopped

4 teaspoons (20 ml) grated fresh ginger*

3 cups (720 ml) chicken broth or water

2 1/2 to 3 pounds (about 6 cups or 1.1 to 1.3 kilograms) butternut or kabocha squash, peeled and cut into 1/2-inch (13 mm) cubes*

2 sweet apples such as Fuji, peeled, cored, and diced

1/2 teaspoon (2.5 ml) salt

1/2 teaspoon (2.5 ml) ground nutmeg

1/2 to 3/4 cup (120 to 178 ml) apple cider

Freshly ground pepper

1/4 cup (60 ml) pumpkin seeds, hulled and toasted*

Antioxidant-rich butternut squash makes a silky soup, garnished here with pumpkin seeds, high in zinc. For a shortcut, look for precut butternut squash, which you may find in the refrigerated section of the produce department. To toast the pumpkin seeds, place them on a baking sheet and bake at 350°F (180°C) until fragrant and slightly brown at the edges, 6 to 8 minutes. To make this a vegetarian dish, use water or vegetable broth in place of chicken broth.

Serves 4

1. Heat the oil in a large pot over medium heat. Add the onion and cook until softened but not browned, about 5 minutes. Add the ginger and stir frequently until fragrant, 1 to 2 minutes.

2. Add the broth, squash, apples, salt, and nutmeg. Adjust the heat to maintain a gentle simmer, cover, and cook until the squash and apples mash easily with a fork, 15 to 20 minutes.

3. Purée the soup in a blender or food processor, in batches if necessary, until smooth. (Be careful because hot liquids may splatter.) Return the soup to the pot and heat gently, thinning with the apple cider.

4. Season to taste with pepper and additional salt, if desired. Ladle into bowls and top each with 1 tablespoon (15 ml) pumpkin seeds.

FERTILITY FACT:
Pumpkin seeds are a great source of the mineral zinc, which is important for testosterone and semen production.

Rice Salad with Salmon and Summer Vegetables

This flavorful brown rice version of the French salade niçoise makes a hearty picnic salad and is a good way to get your fiber, calcium, omega-3s, and folate in a sigle dish.

Serves 4

1. Place the eggs in a saucepan and cover with cold water. Bring the water to a boil over medium heat. Remove from the heat, cover, and let stand for 12 minutes. Carefully remove the eggs with a slotted spoon and place in a bowl of cold water until cool enough to shell, coarsely chop, and set aside.

2. Place the rice in a strainer and rinse under cold running water. In a small saucepan, bring 1³/4 cups (418 ml) water to a boil over medium heat. Add the rice, reduce the heat to maintain a low simmer, and cover. Cook until the water is absorbed and the rice is tender, 35 to 40 minutes. Spoon the rice into a large bowl and let cool.

3. While the rice cooks, trim the ends of the green beans and cut them into 2-inch (50 mm) lengths. Bring a small saucepan of water to a boil and add the beans. Boil until the beans are just crisp-tender, 3 to 5 minutes. Remove from the water with a slotted spoon and rinse under cold running water to cool.

4. Add the beans to the rice along with all of the remaining ingredients. Mix well and season generously with salt and pepper. Serve immediately or cover and chill for up to 1 day. Bring to room temperature before serving.

*3 eggs**

*1 cup (240 ml) short-grain brown rice**

*4 ounces (112 grams) green beans**

*Two 6-ounce (170 gram) cans wild pink salmon, skin and bones removed**

*1 cup (240 ml) cherry tomatoes, halved (6 ounces)**

1/3 cup (80 ml) pitted and coarsely chopped black or green olives

1/4 cup (60 ml) finely chopped red onion

3 tablespoons (45 ml) olive oil

2 tablespoons (30 ml) red wine vinegar

2 tablespoons (30 ml) chopped fresh parsley leaves

Sea salt

Freshly ground pepper

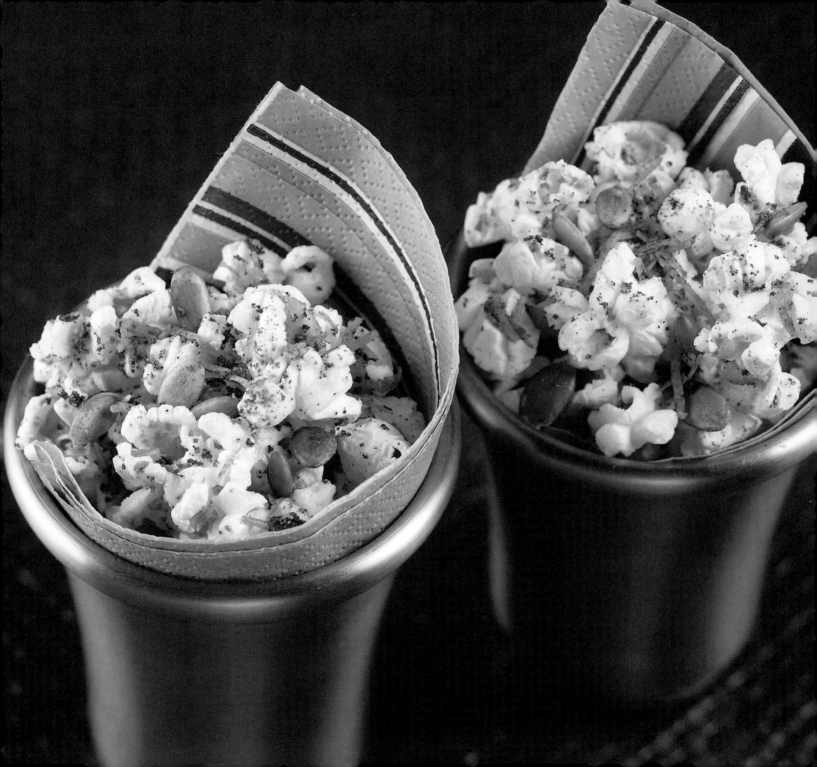

SANDWICHES & SNACKS

The middle of the day provides lots of opportunities for snacks and small meals. Just make sure to take advantage of the best nutrients for fertility. In this chapter, you'll find ideas for smart snacking. For lunch, instead of eating out or skipping lunch altogether, pack up a Turkey–Cream Cheese Wrap. When it comes to between-meal snacking, take the edge off your hunger with a handful of Honey-Sesame Almonds or Parmesan Cheese Popcorn. Fill your pantry with the ingredients for the recipes in this chapter, and you won't be tempted to snack on junk foods or empty calories in the middle of the day.

Turkey–Cream Cheese Wrap

1 piece whole-wheat lavash bread (about 10 by 13 inches, or 254 by 330 mm)*

2 ounces (56 grams) cream cheese at room temperature*

2 tablespoons (30 ml) mango chutney

4 ounces (113 grams) turkey breast, cut into thin slices*

1/4 cup (60 ml), red onion thinly sliced

1/2 cup (120 ml), cucumber thinly sliced

2 handfuls baby spinach leaves (about 1 ounce or 28 grams), washed*

Turkey is a great source of iron and B vitamins. Use leftover turkey or buy roasted turkey breast from the deli rather than using processed packaged turkey meat for these wraps. You can substitute whole-wheat pita bread for the lavash, if you like; simply separate the pita halves, spread the cream cheese and chutney on the inside, and then tuck the rest of the ingredients into the sandwich. For the best results, make sure the cream cheese is slightly softened before you spread it.

Makes 2 sandwiches

1. Place the lavash on a sheet of wax paper. With a flexible spatula or a knife, spread the cream cheese in a thin, even layer over the entire surface of the bread. Spread the mango chutney evenly over the cream cheese. Arrange the turkey evenly over the lavash, leaving a 1-inch (25 mm) border along the short end of the bread. Arrange the onion, cucumber, and spinach evenly over the turkey.

2. Beginning at a short end, roll the lavash as tightly as possible, taking care not to push the filling forward as you go. Chill in the refrigerator for 1 hour, then slice the roll in half on the diagonal and wrap each half tightly in wax paper, if desired. The wrapped sandwiches will keep in the refrigerator for up to 1 day.

FERTILITY FACT:
Do a balancing act with your food for maximum fertility. Try to get one-third of your calories from protein, one-third from complex carbohydrates, and one-third from healthy fats.

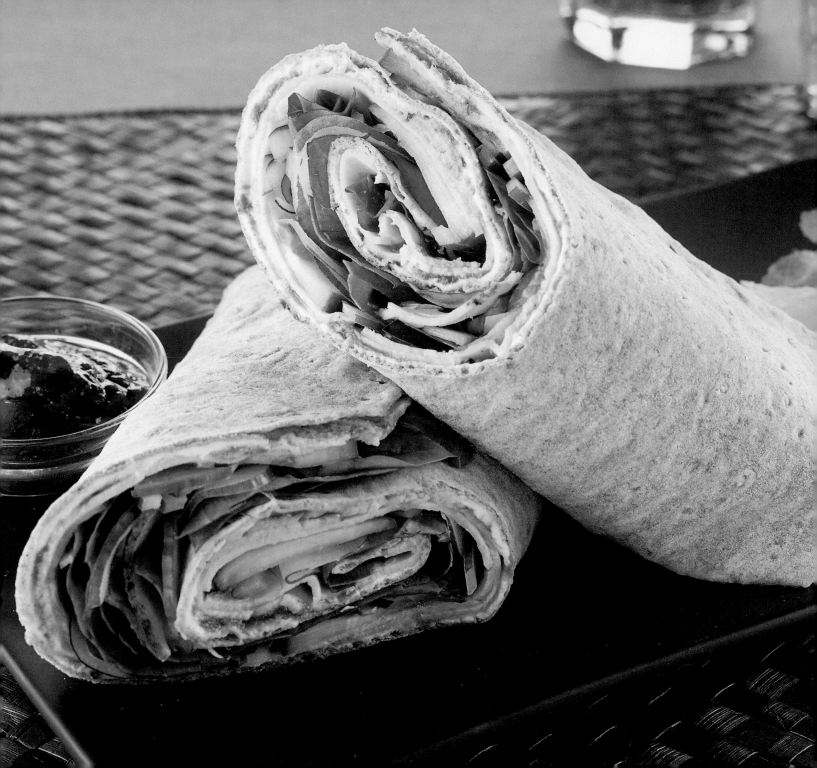

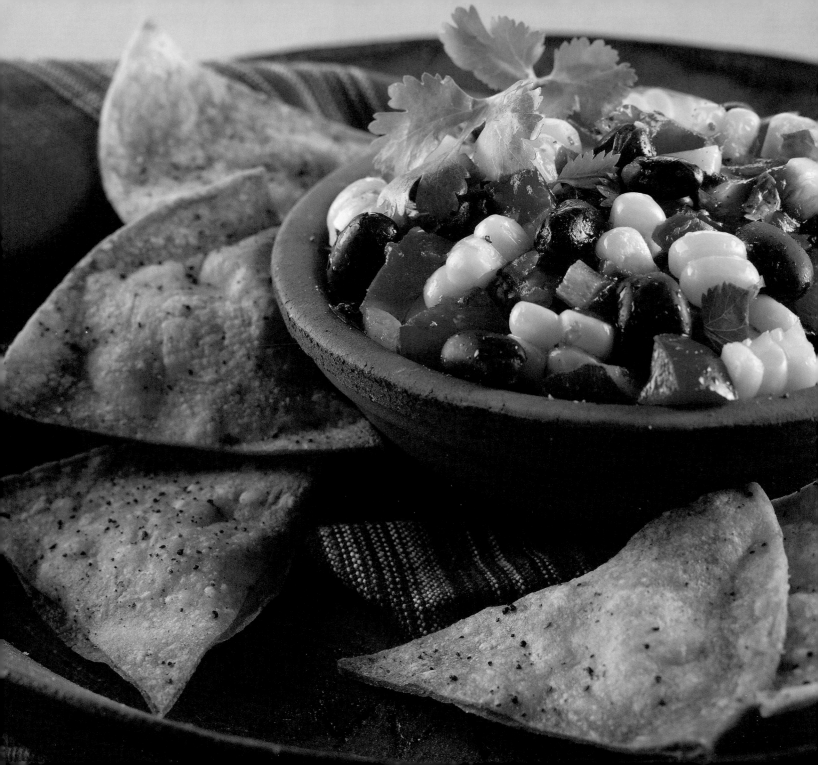

Corn and Black Bean Salsa & Baked Corn Tortilla Chips

Black beans give this hearty salsa fiber as well as nonheme iron. Serve it with the Baked Corn Tortilla Chips or alongside a simple quesadilla. Homemade baked chips have less saturated fat and calories than packaged chips.

Corn and Black Bean Salsa

Serves 4 to 6; makes 4 cups (.95 liter)

In a medium bowl, gently mix the corn, beans, red pepper, onion, cilantro, jalapeño, cinnamon, salsa, olive oil, and lime juice until well combined. Add salt and pepper to taste. Cover and chill for at least 1 hour and up to 2 days. Season to taste with additional lime juice, salt, and pepper, if desired, before serving.

Baked Corn Tortilla Chips

Serves 4

1. Preheat the oven to 375°F (190°C). Lightly oil a baking sheet.

2. Brush one side of each tortilla lightly with olive oil. In a small bowl, mix the chili powder and salt. Stack the tortillas and cut the stack into 6 wedges. Arrange the wedges in a single layer on the baking sheet. Sprinkle with the chili powder mixture. Bake until the tortillas are crisp and dry, approximately 20 minutes. Let cool completely and store in an airtight container for up to 1 week.

For Corn and Black Bean Salsa

1 cup (240 ml) corn kernels, cooked

1 can (15 ounces or 425 grams) black beans, rinsed well and drained*

1 red bell pepper, diced

1/2 small red onion, diced

1/4 cup (60 ml) chopped fresh cilantro

1 jalapeño chile, seeded and chopped

1 tsp. ground cinnamon*

2/3 cup (150 ml) prepared fresh tomato salsa

2 tablespoons (30 ml) olive oil

2 tablespoons (30 ml) fresh lime juice

Salt

Freshly ground pepper

Baked Corn Tortilla Chips

2 1/2 teaspons (12.5 ml) olive oil, or olive oil spray, plus more for greasing

Six 6-inch corn tortillas

1/2 teaspoon (2.5 ml) chili powder

1/2 teaspoon (2.5 ml) salt

Lemony Hummus

1 can (15 ounces or 425 grams)
chickpeas (garbanzo beans),
drained, liquid reserved*

2 tablespoons (30 ml) olive oil

2 teaspoons (10 ml) tahini*

1 teaspoon (5 ml)
ground cumin

1/2 teaspoon (2.5 ml) salt

1/4 teaspoon (1.25 ml) paprika

1/4 teaspoon (1.25 ml)
cayenne pepper

1 lemon, juiced

Hummus is a great source of folate and calcium. If you have a blender or a food processor, in just a few minutes you can make hummus that's as delicious as any you can buy, if not more so, at a fraction of the cost. Even more important, you can be sure of the quality of the ingredients that go into it.

Tahini is a creamy purée of toasted sesame seeds. If you can't find it, you can leave it out and still have a tasty chickpea dip. Feel free to double this recipe and use it for sandwiches or wraps, or for dipping fresh vegetables or baked pita chips.

Serves 4 to 6; makes 1¼ cups (300 ml)

In a blender or food processor, whirl the chickpeas, oil, tahini, cumin, salt, paprika, cayenne, and lemon juice until smooth. Add the reserved chickpea liquid as needed to make a smooth purée. Transfer to an airtight container and refrigerate for up to 3 days.

Avocado-Yogurt Dip

Avocados contain more folate per ounce than any other fruit. This tasty guacamole dip is fortified with yogurt, which serves the dual purpose of adding much-needed calcium and cutting down slightly on the calories and fat. It's wonderful for dipping raw carrot and red bell pepper sticks, or Baked Corn Tortilla Chips (page 77).

Serves 6 to 8; makes about 2 cups (480 ml)

Cut the avocados in half and scoop out the pits. Remove the flesh from the peel and coarsely chop. Place all of the ingredients except for the jalapeño in a blender or food processor and pulse until smooth. Transfer to a bowl and stir in the jalapeño to taste. Stir in more lime juice and salt to taste, if desired.

2 ripe avocados*

1/2 cup (120 ml) plain whole-milk yogurt*

1/3 cup (80 ml) chopped red onion

2 tablespoons (30 ml) chopped fresh cilantro

1 1/2 tablespoons (22.5 ml) fresh lime juice

2 teaspoons (10 ml) ground cumin

1 clove garlic, minced

1/4 teaspoon (1.25 ml) sea salt

1 to 1 1/2 teaspoons (5 to 7.5 ml) seeded and finely chopped jalapeño chile

FERTILITY FACT:

Fat isn't always bad. Monounsaturated fat, such as the fat in avocados, can actually help improve your chances of conceiving because it reduces inflammation and insulin sensitivity, two factors that can disrupt hormone balance in the body.

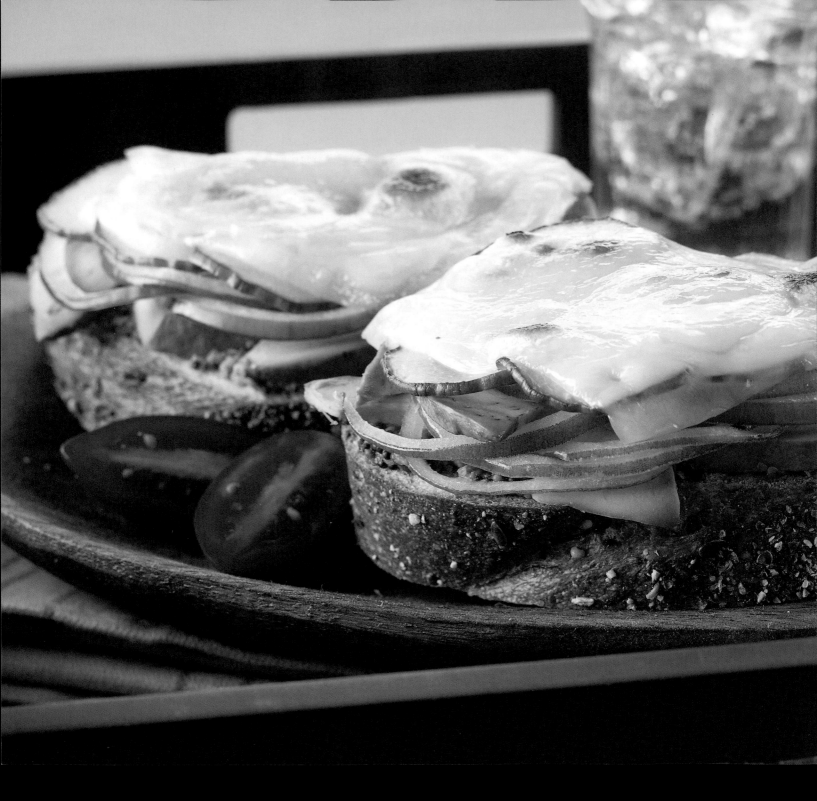

Open-Faced Veggie Melt

You'll want to keep the ingredients for this quick, tasty sandwich on your regular shopping list, since it gives you whole-grain carbohydrates, folate, and calcium in one simple dish. Use half an avocado for this sandwich at lunch, and chop the remaining half into a salad for dinner. Or wrap it well and refrigerate it to use the next day. You can easily turn this knife-and-fork melt into a great sandwich to go—just top it with a second slice of bread.

Serves 1

1. Preheat the broiler.

2. Spread the bread generously with mustard. Scoop the avocado flesh from the peel with a spoon and slice lengthwise. Fan the avocado on the bread. Arrange the onion slices and cucumber over the avocado and sprinkle lightly with salt and pepper. Top with the cheese.

3. Place under the broiler until the cheese is just melted and bubbling, about 1 minute.

1 slice hearty, whole-grain bread*

Whole-grain Dijon mustard

1/2 ripe avocado*

1 to 2 thin slices red onion

4 to 6 thin slices cucumber

Sea salt

Freshly ground pepper

1 slice (about 1 ounce or 28 grams) Swiss cheese*

Parmesan Cheese Popcorn

3 tablespoons (45 ml)
finely grated
Parmesan cheese

1 teaspoon (5 ml)
smoked paprika

¼ teaspoon (1.25 ml)
ground cumin

¼ teaspoon (1.25 ml) sea salt

6 cups (1.4 liters)
popped plain popcorn*

¼ cup (60 ml)
pumpkin seeds, toasted
(see page 70)*

1½ tablespoons (23 ml) butter

With its addition of sea salt, cumin, and zinc-rich pumpkin seeds, this tasty popcorn is perfect for times when you feel like crunching on something light and salty.

Serves 4, makes 6 cups (1.4 liters)

1. In a small bowl, combine the cheese, paprika, cumin, and sea salt. Place the popcorn and pumpkin seeds in a large bowl.

2. Melt butter in a small skillet over low heat. Drizzle the popcorn and pumpkin seeds with the butter and toss well with the Parmesan cheese mixture. Serve immediately.

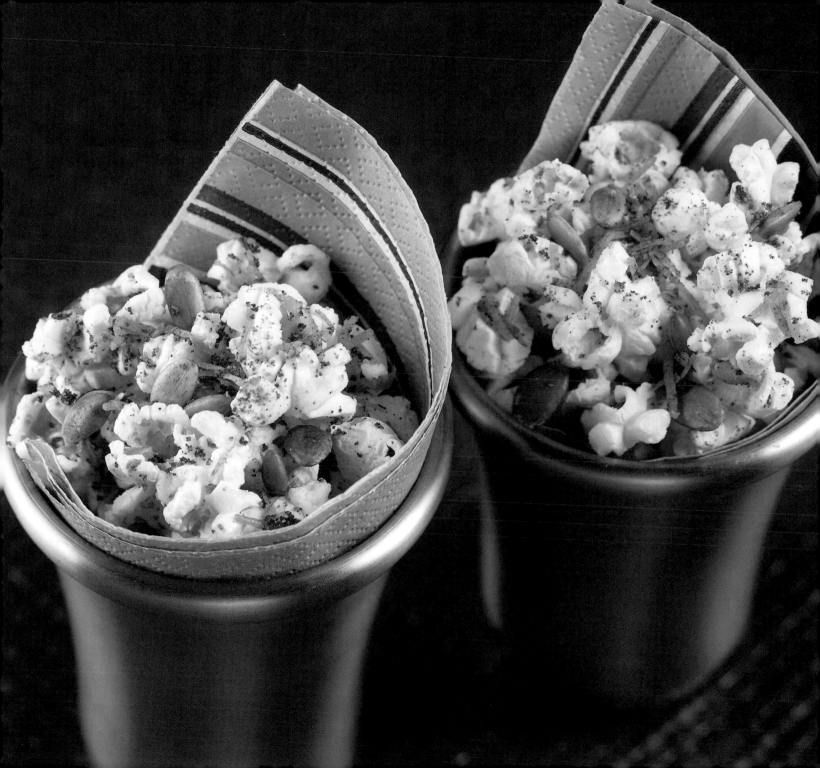

Toasted Cheese Sandwich with Red Peppers and Pesto

*2 slices
(about 1/2 inch or
12.7 mm thick)
whole-wheat sourdough
or crusty artisan-style
whole-grain bread**

*1 tablespoon (15 ml)
purchased pesto sauce**

*1 ounce (28 grams) mozzarella
cheese, cut into slices**

1/2 roasted red bell pepper, sliced

Whole-wheat sourdough makes a delicious toasted cheese sandwich, particularly when you add a few roasted bell pepper slices and a spoonful of pesto. Look for roasted bell peppers in jars in the pickle aisle of the supermarket. They make a sweet and vitamin-rich sandwich filling.

Serves 1

Preheat the broiler. Toast the bread on one side. Remove from under the broiler, spread each untoasted side with pesto sauce, and top with cheese. Return to the broiler just until the cheese is melted. Place the pepper slices on one slice of the bread, and sandwich the two slices together.

FERTILITY FACT:
Trans fats contained in hydrogenated or partially hydrogenated oils can sabotage fertility. Experts theorize they may interfere with ovulation. So read labels carefully, especially when buying packaged bread, crackers, cookies, and other baked goods.

Spinach and Three-Cheese Calzones

Bake a batch of these spinach-packed pies on the weekend, freeze or refrigerate, and pair them with fresh fruit for meatless weekday lunches that are full of calcium and iron. You can make your own dough from the recipe on page 107, or use purchased whole-wheat pizza dough, available in the freezer or refrigerated sections of many markets.

Serves 4

1. Heat the oil in a large frying pan over medium-high heat. Add the garlic and stir until fragrant but not brown, about 45 seconds. Add the spinach leaves (if it looks like too much spinach for the pan, keep adding spinach gradually as the leaves cook and shrink down) and cook, stirring frequently until wilted, 2 to 3 minutes. Transfer to a colander and let cool. When cool enough to handle, squeeze as much liquid as possible from the leaves, and then coarsely chop.

2. In a medium bowl, stir together the cheeses, olives (if using), egg yolk, red pepper flakes, and spinach until well blended.

3. On a lightly floured surface, cut the pizza dough into 4 equal pieces. Gently stretch and press each piece (or roll with a lightly floured rolling pin) into an 8-inch (203 mm) round. Mound the filling evenly on one half of each of the 4 rounds of dough. Fold each round in half to enclose the filling. Fold and pinch the edges together to seal. Transfer the calzones to a baking sheet.

4. In a small bowl, beat the egg white lightly with 1 tablespoon (15 ml) water. Brush the tops of the calzones lightly with the egg white mixture and sprinkle with the sesame seeds. Bake until the calzones are golden brown, 15 to 18 minutes. Let cool on the baking sheet.

1 tablespoon (15 ml) extra-virgin olive oil

1 clove garlic, minced

10 ounces (280 grams) baby spinach leaves (about 5 cups packed) washed*

1 cup (240 ml) whole-milk ricotta*

3/4 cup (178 ml) shredded whole-milk mozzarella*

1/4 cup (60 ml) grated Parmesan cheese

1/4 cup (60 ml) chopped pitted kalamata olives (optional)

1 large egg, separated

1/4 teaspoon (1 ml) crushed red pepper flakes

1 pound (454 grams) whole-wheat pizza dough (see note), at room temperature*

1 teaspoon (5 ml) sesame seeds*

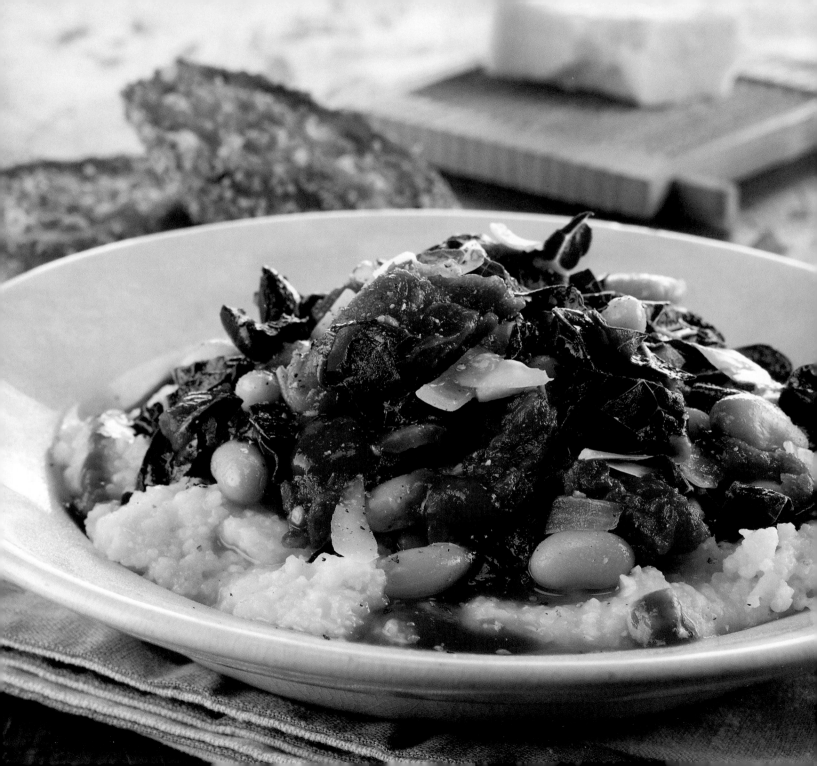

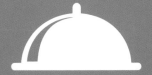

MAIN DISHES

When it comes to the main course, you have many opportunities to incorporate nutrients that support conception. Since protein and iron from plant sources have been linked to a reduced risk of ovulatory infertility, in this chapter we've included recipes for tasty meatless dishes like Southwest Vegetable Chili and Barley-Mushroom Risotto that take advantage of fiber- and protein-rich beans, whole grains, and vegetables. Not everyone eats meatless meals every night, so we've also included dishes that feature lean, vitamin B- and iron-rich protein along with vegetables: dishes like Grilled Chicken Fajitas and whole-wheat Linguine with Turkey Bolognese. Fish is one of the richest sources of fertility-friendly omega-3s, and you'll find it here, too, in dishes like Maple-Glazed Salmon and Penne with Salmon, Peas, and Asparagus.

Barley Mushroom Risotto

6¹/₂ to 7 cups (1.4 liters)
vegetable broth

1¹/₂ tablespoons (22.5 ml) olive oil

1 cup (240 ml) leeks
(white and pale green parts only),
cut into thin slices, rinsed well*

1 clove garlic, minced

4 cups sliced fresh mixed
mushrooms (about 12 ounces
or 336 grams)*

¹/₂ teaspoon (2.5 ml)
dried thyme, or
1 teaspoon (5 ml)
fresh thyme leaves

¹/₄ teaspoon (1.25 ml) salt

Freshly ground pepper

1 cup (240 ml) pearl barley*

¹/₂ cup (120ml)
grated Parmesan cheese

2 tablespoons (30 ml)
chopped fresh parsley

This hearty meatless main dish pairs selenium-rich mushrooms with chewy, nutty barley for a filling, fiber-rich meal. When preparing the leeks, it's easiest to wash them after you slice them; just place them in a colander and rinse under running water until free of grit.

Serves 4

1. Bring the broth to a simmer in a medium saucepan over medium-high heat. Turn off the heat and cover to keep warm.

2. Heat the oil in a large saucepan over medium heat. Add the leeks and garlic and cook, stirring frequently, until the leeks are soft, 5 to 6 minutes. Add the mushrooms, thyme, salt, and a few grinds of pepper. Cook, stirring frequently, until the mushrooms soften and start to brown, 4 to 5 minutes.

3. Add 5 ¹/₂ cups (1.2 liters) of the hot broth and the barley. Cover and simmer over medium-low heat, stirring occasionally and adding more broth, ¹/₂ cup (60 ml) at a time, as it is absorbed by the barley. Cook until the barley is tender, about 50 to 55 minutes.

4. Stir in the Parmesan cheese and parsley. Season to taste with additional salt and pepper, if desired.

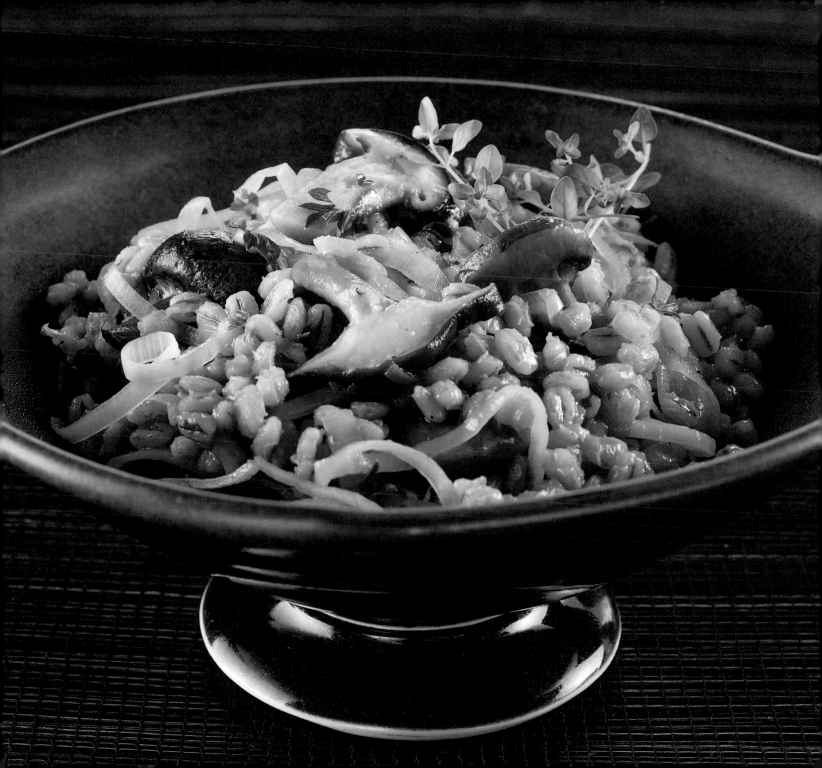

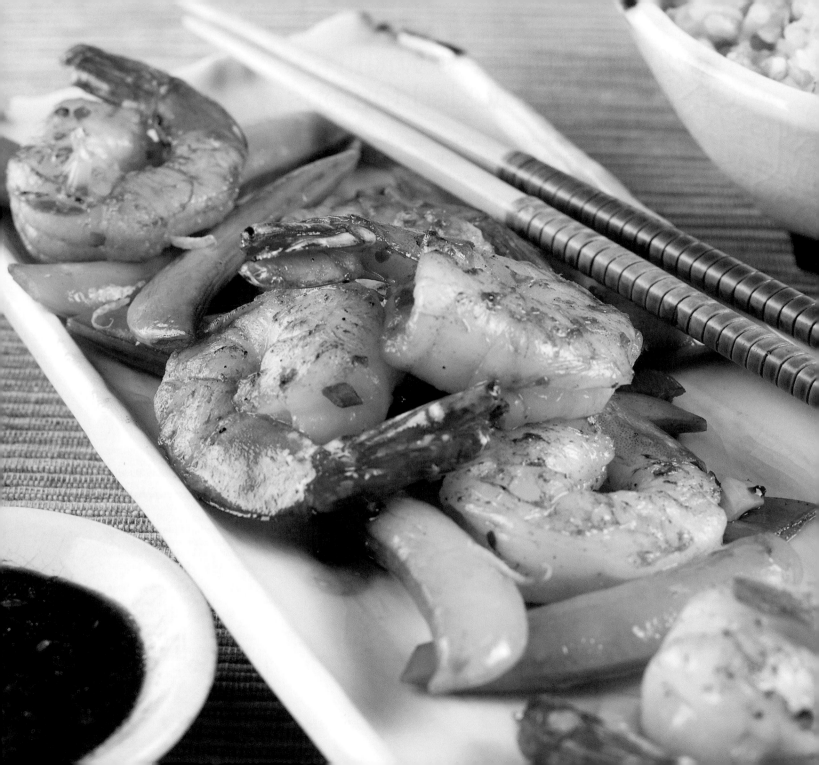

Citrus Shrimp with Sugar Snap Peas

Shrimp are a low-calorie source of protein, iron, zinc, and B vitamins. Pair them with folate-rich snap peas in this quick stir-fry. If the shrimp you're using were previously frozen, drain them well and pat them dry with a paper towel before adding them to the marinade. If you can't find sugar snap peas, you can substitute snow peas.

Serves 4

1. In a bowl large enough to hold the shrimp, mix the soy sauce, ginger, orange zest, garlic, and red pepper flakes. Add the shrimp and mix to coat. Refrigerate for 15 minutes.

2. In a large frying pan, heat the oil over high heat. Add the shrimp mixture, green onions, and snap peas. Stir until the shrimp are evenly pink and cooked in the center, about 2 minutes. Add the broth and orange juice and cook to reduce the sauce slightly, about 1 minute longer.

2 tablespoons (30 ml) soy sauce

1 tablespoon (15 ml) minced peeled fresh ginger

1 teaspoon (5 ml) minced orange zest

1 clove garlic, minced

1/4 teaspoon (1 ml) crushed red pepper flakes

1 pound (454 grams) uncooked large shrimp, peeled and deveined*

1 1/2 tablespoons (22.5 ml) canola oil

4 green onions, cut into thin slices

1 pound (454 grams) sugar snap peas, ends trimmed and strings removed*

1/4 cup (60 ml) chicken broth

2 tablespoons (30 ml) fresh orange juice

FERTILITY FACT:

Soy sauce and other foods containing soy are okay in moderation when trying to conceive. But women should try to avoid soy around the time of ovulation, because it may sabotage sperm cells swimming in the female reproductive tract trying to fertilize an egg. Men should keep soy intake low so it won't affect sperm quality.

Pumpkin Macaroni and Cheese

1 slice sturdy white bread
(about 1 ounce or 28 grams),
crusts removed

1/2 cup (120 ml) grated
Parmesan cheese, divided

1 can (15 ounces or 425 grams)
pumpkin purée*

1 cup (240 ml) chicken broth

12 ounces (336 grams) dried
whole-wheat pasta shells*

1 1/2 tablespoons (22.5 ml) butter

1/2 cup (120 ml) minced onion

1 1/2 tablespoons (22.5 ml)
all-purpose flour

1 cup (240 ml) whole milk*

2 cups (480 ml) shredded Gouda
cheese, divided*

1/2 teaspoon (2.5 ml) salt

1/8 teaspoon (.5 ml)
ground nutmeg

1/8 teaspoon (.5 ml)
cayenne pepper

A creamy sauce of cheese and pumpkin clings to whole-wheat pasta shells in this new take on a classic comfort dish. Pumpkin is rich in antioxidants, and milk adds calcium and protein, plus the fertility benefits of whole milk dairy. Steamed broccoli makes a great side dish.

Serves 4 to 6

1. Preheat the oven to 350°F (180°C). Tear the bread into chunks and whirl in a blender until fine crumbs form. Mix with half of the Parmesan cheese and set aside.

2. In a small saucepan, over medium heat stir the pumpkin purée and broth together. Bring to a simmer, stirring occasionally. Cover and keep warm.

3. Bring a large pot of lightly salted water to a boil. Add the pasta and cook until al dente, 8 to 10 minutes. Drain well and pour into a 2-quart baking dish.

4. Melt the butter in a large pot or Dutch oven over medium heat. Add the onion and cook, stirring frequently, until softened but not browned, about 5 minutes. Stir in the flour and cook for another minute. Slowly whisk in the milk and bring the mixture to a simmer; cook, whisking frequently, until the sauce thickens, about 3 minutes. Remove from the heat.

5. Stir in half of the Gouda, the remaining Parmesan, and the salt, nutmeg, and cayenne, and whisk vigorously until melted and smooth. Slowly pour in the pumpkin mixture, whisking until well blended.

6. Pour the pumpkin-cheese sauce over the pasta and stir gently to coat. Sprinkle with the remaining Gouda and then the breadcrumb mixture. Bake until the crumbs are golden, about 20 minutes.

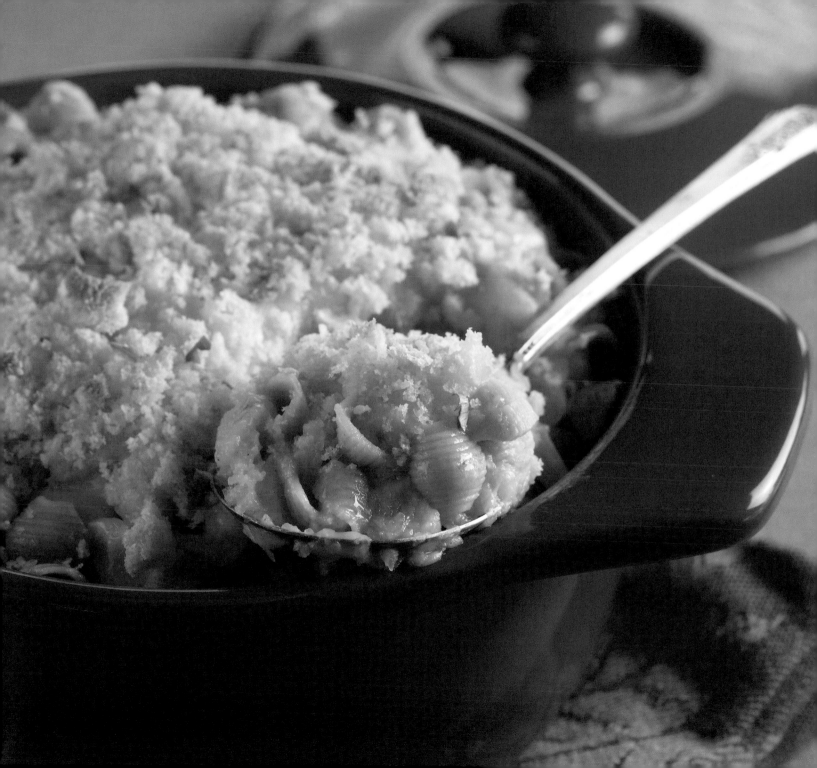

Linguine with Turkey Bolognese

2 tablespoons (30 ml) olive oil

1 yellow onion, finely chopped

1 carrot, peeled and finely chopped

1 stalk celery, finely chopped

2 cloves garlic, peeled and minced

1 pound (454 grams) ground turkey leg and thigh meat*

1 can (28 ounces or 800 grams) crushed or puréed tomatoes*

1/4 cup (60 ml) red wine

1 teaspoon (5 ml) dried oregano

1/4 teaspoon (1.25 ml) salt

1/4 teaspoon (1.25 ml) pepper

1/8 teaspoon (.5 ml) ground nutmeg

1 pound (454 grams) whole-wheat linguine

Grated Parmesan cheese for serving

Ground turkey adds iron, B vitamins, selenium, and protein to this thick, lycopene-rich sauce, which tops whole-wheat linguine. If you have a bit of Parmesan cheese rind in the refrigerator, add it to the sauce as it simmers. And, if you prefer not to cook with wine, feel free to substitute 1/4 cup (60 ml) chicken broth.

Serves 6

1. Heat the oil in a large pot or Dutch oven over medium heat. Add the onion, carrot, celery, and garlic. Cook, stirring frequently and reducing heat as necessary, until the vegetables are softened but not browned, about 5 minutes. Add the turkey, breaking up the meat with a wooden spoon, and cook until no longer pink, 5 to 7 minutes.

2. Add the tomatoes, wine, oregano, salt, pepper, and nutmeg. Adjust the heat to maintain a gentle simmer, cover, and cook, stirring occasionally, until the mixture is a thick, dark red sauce, 20 to 25 minutes.

3. Bring a large pot of lightly salted water to a boil. Cook the linguine until just al dente, 9 to 11 minutes. Drain well and toss with the sauce. Serve with the Parmesan cheese for sprinkling over the top.

Penne with Salmon, Peas, and Asparagus

A bit of cream stirred in at the end adds a silky, rounded flavor to this spring pasta dish, which is loaded with folate, iron, protein, and omega-3s. Ask your grocer to skin the salmon fillet for you and remove the tiny bones.

Serves 4

1. Preheat the oven to 400°F (200°C). Place the salmon in a baking pan and drizzle with about 1 tablespoon (15 ml) olive oil. Sprinkle generously with salt and pepper. Bake until no longer opaque in the center, 12 to 15 minutes.

2. Trim the stem ends from the asparagus and cut on the diagonal into 2-inch (50 mm) lengths.

3. Bring a large pot of lightly salted water to a boil. Add the penne and boil for 8 minutes. Add the asparagus to the water and cook for 2 minutes. Add the peas and cook for 1 minute, or until the pasta is al dente. Drain the pasta and vegetables and return to the pot. Stir in the lemon juice, lemon zest, and the salmon, using a fork to break up the salmon into bite-size pieces. Season to taste with salt and pepper. Stir in the basil and cream and serve immediately.

1 pound (454 grams) salmon fillet, skin and bones removed*

1 tablespoon (15 ml) olive oil

Salt

Pepper

1/2 pound (224 grams) asparagus*

12 ounces (336 grams) whole-wheat penne*

1 1/2 cups (360 ml) fresh or frozen shelled green peas (about 8 ounces or 227 grams; no need to thaw if frozen)*

3 tablespoons (45 ml) fresh lemon juice

1 tablespoon (15 ml) grated lemon zest

1/4 cup (60 ml) torn basil leaves*

1/4 cup (60 ml) cream

FERTILITY FACT:

Some fish contain high levels of mercury, which can be harmful to an unborn child even when eaten up to a year before conception. But wild salmon, shrimp, pollock, catfish, and canned light tuna are all low in mercury.

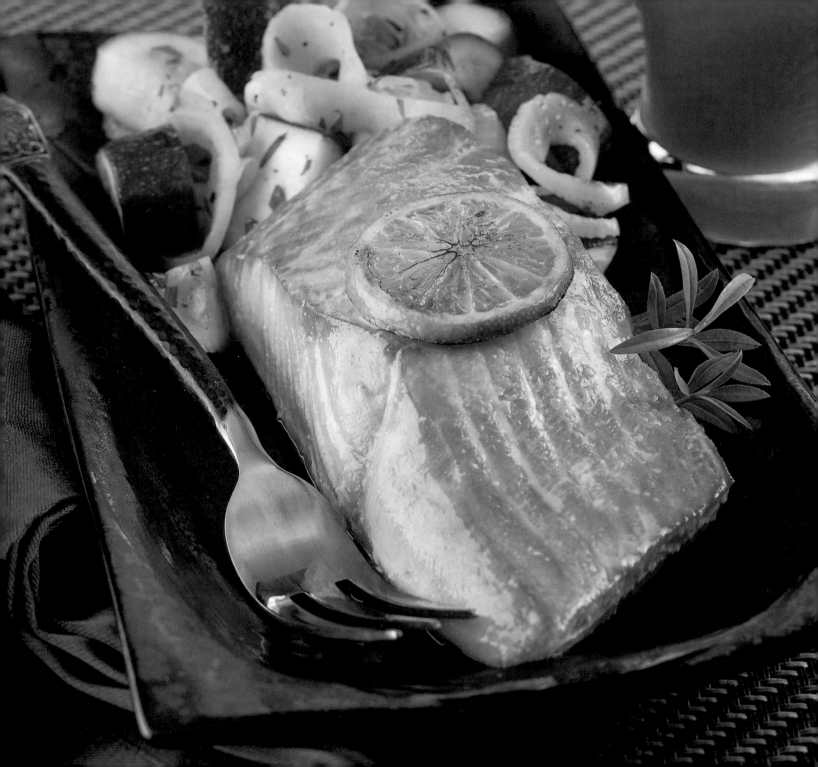

Maple-Glazed Salmon

This is a simple and delicious way to prepare salmon, a great source of protein and omega-3s that has B vitamins, too. Ask your grocer to skin the fillet and remove the pin bones. Also, use Grade B maple syrup; it is thicker and more flavorful than Grade A. Good sides to serve with this dish are Wilted Spinach with Garlic (page 155) and Mashed Sweet Potatoes with Yogurt and Lime (page 154).

Serves 4

1. Preheat the oven to 400°F (200°C). Line a shallow baking pan with foil.

2. In a small bowl, mix the maple syrup, lime juice, mustard, and salt. Reserve 1 tablespoon (15 ml) of the mixture.

3. Place the salmon, skinned side down, on the prepared pan. Brush the salmon with half of the syrup mixture.

4. Bake the salmon in the middle of the oven for 8 minutes. Switch the oven to the broiler setting and brush the salmon with the remaining syrup mixture. Broil the salmon 4 to 5 inches from the heat until just cooked through, 3 to 5 minutes. Drizzle the fish with the reserved tablespoon of glaze mixture just before serving.

3 tablespoons (45 ml) Grade B maple syrup

1 tablespoon (15 ml) fresh lime juice

1 1/2 teaspoons (7.5 ml) Dijon mustard

1/2 teaspoon (2.5 ml) salt

1 1/2 pounds (681 grams) salmon fillet, about 1 inch (25 mm) thick, cut into 4 pieces, skin and bones removed*

Stir-Fried Pork with Bell Peppers and Basil

1 pound (454 grams) pork tenderloin*

½ cup (120 ml) chicken broth

3 tablespoons (45 ml) low-sodium soy sauce

3 tablespoons (45 ml) honey

¼ cup (60 ml) fresh lime juice

2 tablespoons (30 ml) canola oil, divided

2 medium red bell peppers, thinly sliced*

½ cup (120 ml) thinly sliced shallots or red onion

½ cup (120 ml) roughly torn basil leaves

Stir-fries, because they cook quickly, are great ways to combine a modest portion of lean meat with lots of fresh, vitamin packed vegetables. The pork in this dish is a good source of vitamin B-12. Serve it over steamed brown rice.

Serves 4

1. Trim the silvery membrane from the pork; cut into thin slices across the grain.

2. In a small bowl, mix the broth, soy sauce, honey, and lime juice; set aside.

3. Heat 1 tablespoon (15 ml) of the oil in a large frying pan over high heat. When hot, add the bell peppers and stir until softened, 2 to 3 minutes. Transfer the bell peppers to a plate and add the remaining tablespoon of oil to the pan. Add the shallots and cook, stirring constantly, until fragrant but not brown, about 45 seconds. Add the pork and stir frequently until no longer pink, 3 to 5 minutes. Return the bell peppers to the pan and stir in the broth mixture and the basil. Cook about 1 minute to heat through.

FERTILITY FACT:

A little-known nutrient called *carnitine*, contained in meat, helps improve sperm quality and motility.

Scallops with Summer Vegetable Succotash

Scallops are a low-calorie, low-fat source of protein and zinc. They cook quickly, making them ideal for weeknight meals like this one. The colorful mix of vegetables here adds vitamins and antioxidants.

Serves 4

1. Heat 1 tablespoon (15 ml) of the oil in a large frying pan over medium-high heat. Add the onion and stir frequently until softened but not browned, about 3 minutes. Add the bell pepper and zucchini and cook, stirring frequently, until the vegetables soften, 2 to 4 minutes. Add the corn and cook 2 minutes more. Sprinkle mixture with salt and pepper. Add the vinegar and stir for 1 minute. Pour the vegetables into a large bowl and stir in the parsley. Wipe out the pan with a paper towel.

2. Pat the scallops dry with another paper towel and sprinkle them with salt and pepper. Heat the remaining tablespoon of oil over medium-high heat. Add the scallops and cook, turning once, until browned on both sides and just cooked in the center, 4 to 6 minutes total.

3. Spoon the vegetables onto plates and top evenly with scallops. Serve immediately.

2 tablespoons (30 ml) olive oil, divided

1/4 cup (60 ml) finely chopped red onion

1 red bell pepper, diced*

2 small zucchini (about 8 ounces or 227 grams), diced*

1 cup (240 ml) fresh corn kernels*

Sea salt

Freshly ground pepper

1 1/2 teaspoons (7.5 ml) red wine vinegar

2 tablespoons (30 ml) chopped fresh parsley

1 1/4 pounds (567 grams) scallops (each 1 1/2 to 2 inches or 38 to 50 mm wide)*

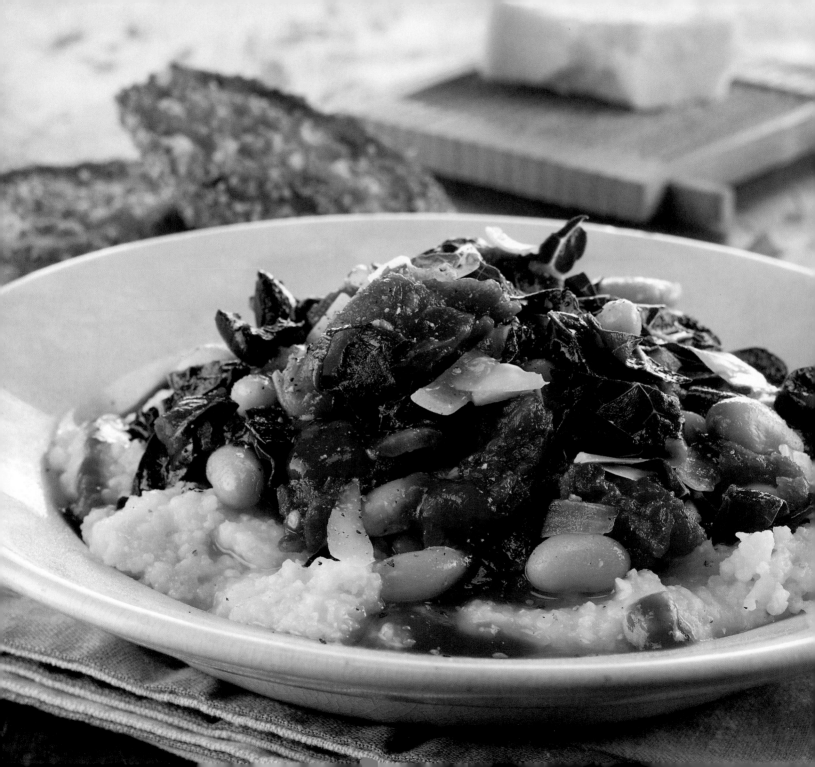

Kale and White Bean Ragout with Parmesan Polenta

Calcium-rich dinosaur kale, also known as Lacinato kale, and white beans join kalamata olives and lycopene-rich tomatoes in this flavorful dish. If you buy organic canned beans, you can reserve the fiber-rich liquid and add it to the dish. Because this dish contains salty ingredients, you probably won't need to add additional salt.

Serves 4 to 6

1. To make the polenta: Bring 4$^{1}/_2$ cups (1.1 liters) water and the salt to a boil in a medium saucepan over high heat. Whisk in the polenta, reduce the heat to medium-low and simmer, stirring occasionally, until polenta is thick and no longer grainy, 25 to 30 minutes. Remove from the heat and stir in the cheese; add pepper to taste. Cover and keep warm.

2. To make the ragout: Tear the kale leaves from the stems and tough center ribs. Rinse the leaves well and cut into $^1/_4$-inch (6 mm) ribbons (discard the ribs and stems).

3. Heat the oil in a large pot or Dutch oven over medium heat. Add the onion and garlic and cook until the onion is softened but not browned, about 5 minutes. Add the tomatoes, including the juices, using a fork to break up the tomatoes into small chunks. Add the beans, including their liquid, $^3/_4$ cup (178 ml) broth, and the kale, cumin, and paprika. Bring to a simmer and cook, uncovered, until the kale is tender, about 15 minutes, adding more broth if the ragout begins to look dry. Stir in the lemon juice and olives. Add pepper to taste. Spoon the polenta onto plates and top with ragout.

Parmesan Polenta

$^1/_2$ teaspoon (2.5 ml) salt

1 cup (240 ml) stone-ground cornmeal (polenta)*

$^1/_3$ cup (80 ml) grated Parmesan cheese

Freshly ground pepper

Ragout

1 bunch (8 to 12 ounces or 227 to 336 grams) dinosaur kale*

2 tablespoons (30 ml) olive oil

1 onion, peeled and finely chopped

2 cloves garlic, peeled and minced

1 can (28 ounces or 800 grams) whole peeled tomatoes*

2 cans (14.5 ounces or 425 grams each) cannellini beans (white kidney beans), not drained*

$^3/_4$ to 1 cup (178 to 240 ml) chicken or vegetable broth

$^1/_2$ teaspoon (2.5 ml) ground cumin

$^1/_2$ teaspoon (2.5 ml) smoked paprika

2 teaspoons (10 ml) fresh lemon juice

3 tablespoons (45 ml) chopped pitted kalamata olives

Pepper

Southwest Vegetable Chili

2 tablespoons (30 ml) olive oil

1 red onion, diced

2 cloves garlic, minced

³⁄4 cup (178 ml) fresh or frozen corn kernels

¹⁄2 cup (120 ml) diced red bell pepper

¹⁄2 cup (120 ml) diced yellow bell pepper

1 tablespoon (15 ml) minced, seeded jalapeño chile

2 tablespoons (30 ml) chili powder

1 teaspoon (5 ml) dried oregano

1 teaspoon (5 ml) ground cumin

¹⁄2 teaspoon (2.5 ml) salt

1 can (28 ounces or 800 grams) diced or crushed tomatoes

2 cans (14.5 ounces or 425 grams each) pinto beans, drained

¹⁄4 cup (60 ml) chopped fresh cilantro

2 teaspoons (10 ml) lime juice

Fiber-rich beans join vitamin-packed vegetables and Southwestern spices in this satisfying vegetarian chili. Any leftovers freeze well for meatless weekday lunches. Serve the chili with cornbread muffins, if you like.

Serves 4 to 6

1. Heat the oil in a large pot over medium-high heat. Add the onion and garlic and stir frequently until onion softens, about 5 minutes. Add corn, peppers, and jalapeño and cook 2 minutes. Stir in the spices and salt and cook for 1 minute more.

2. Add the tomatoes, beans, and ³⁄4 cup (178 ml) water; bring to a boil. Cover, reduce the heat, and simmer for 20 minutes to blend the flavors, stirring occasionally. Stir in the cilantro and lime juice.

FERTILITY FACT:
For women, getting protein from vegetarian sources such as beans, peas, or nuts (rather than from meat) provides some protection against ovulatory infertility.

Roasted Vegetable Pizza

This colorful pie has a whole-wheat crust and lots of vegetables. As a shortcut, you can use a pound of purchased whole-wheat pizza dough, available in the freezer and/or refrigerated sections of many markets.

Makes one 14-inch (356 mm) pizza; serves 6

1. To make the dough: Sprinkle the yeast over $3/4$ cup (178 ml) lukewarm water in a large bowl. Let stand until softened, about 5 minutes. Stir in 1 cup (240 ml) all-purpose flour, the whole-wheat flour, salt, and oil and mix until the dough is moistened and slightly stretchy. Scrape the dough onto a lightly floured board. Knead until smooth, elastic, and no longer sticky; add flour as required to prevent sticking. (If using a mixer with a dough hook, beat on high speed until dough is smooth and elastic but still a little sticky. If dough still clings to the sides of the bowl, beat in more flour, 2 tablespoons [30 ml] at a time.) Return the dough to the bowl, cover, and let rise at room temperature until doubled, about 1 hour.

2. To make the topping: Preheat the oven to 400°F (200°C). In a large baking pan, mix the squashes, bell pepper, onion, and garlic with 1 tablespoon (15 ml) olive oil, the oregano, salt, and pepper. Bake until the vegetables are soft and lightly browned, stirring once midway through baking time, 18 to 25 minutes. Increase the oven temperature to 500°F (260°C).

3. Oil a 14-inch (356 mm) pizza pan or a large baking sheet and sprinkle lightly with cornmeal. Scrape the dough out onto a lightly floured surface and press gently to expel the air. Stretch the dough (or roll it with a lightly floured rolling pin) to make a 14-inch (356 mm) round about $1/4$ inch (6 mm) thick and place it on the prepared pan. Spoon the sauce evenly over the dough. Top with the cheeses and vegetables.

4. Bake in the lower half of the oven until the crust is browned, 10 to 15 minutes.

Dough

1 envelope (2 teaspoons or 10 ml) active dry yeast

1 to $1^{1}/4$ cups (240 to 300 ml) all-purpose flour

$3/4$ cup (178 ml) whole-wheat flour*

$3/4$ teaspoon (4 ml) salt

1 tablespoon (15 ml) extra-virgin olive oil

Topping

2 medium zucchini, cut into $1/2$-inch-thick (13-mm-thick) slices*

2 yellow crookneck squash, cut into $1/2$-inch-thick (13-mm-thick) slices*

1 red bell pepper, cut into 1-inch chunks

$1/2$ red onion, cut into 1-inch (25 mm) chunks

4 cloves garlic, peeled and smashed

1 tablespoon (15 ml) olive oil, plus more for preparing pan

$1/4$ teaspoon (1 ml) dried oregano

Sea salt

Freshly ground pepper

Cornmeal for preparing pan

$3/4$ cup (178 ml) good-quality purchased tomato or pizza sauce

1 cup (240 ml) shredded mozzarella cheese*

$1/4$ cup (60 ml) Parmesan cheese*

Chicken and Broccoli Stir-Fry with Cashews

6 cups (1.4 liters) broccoli florets,
cut into bite-size pieces*

2 tablespoons (30 ml)
soy sauce, divided

4 green onions, cut into thin slices

2 cloves garlic, minced

1 tablespoon (15 ml)
minced peeled fresh ginger

1/4 teaspoon (1.25 ml)
red pepper flakes (optional)

1 pound (454 grams)
skinless boneless
chicken breast halves
(about 2), cut across the
grain into thin slices*

3/4 cup (178 ml) chicken broth

1 tablespoon (15 ml) cornstarch

1 tablespoon (15 ml) canola oil

1/2 cup (120 ml) toasted cashews*

4 cups (.95 liter) cooked
brown rice*

Ginger and garlic make this bright stir-fry fragrant and flavorful. Serve it with steamed brown rice for a dinner with iron, fiber, B vitamins, and antioxidants.

Serves 4

1. Bring a medium pot of water to a boil. Add the broccoli and cook until crisp-tender, 2 to 4 minutes. Drain well and set aside.

2. In a medium bowl, combine 1 tablespoon (15 ml) of the soy sauce, the onions, garlic, ginger, and red pepper flakes, if using. Add the chicken and turn to coat. Chill for 15 minutes.

3. Combine the chicken broth, cornstarch, and remaining tablespoon soy sauce in a small bowl and set aside.

4. Heat the oil in a large wok or frying pan over high heat. Add the chicken and stir frequently until most of the chicken is opaque, 2 to 3 minutes. Add the broccoli and broth mixture. Cook until the chicken is cooked through and the liquid thickens, 1 to 3 minutes longer. Stir in the cashews and serve immediately over rice.

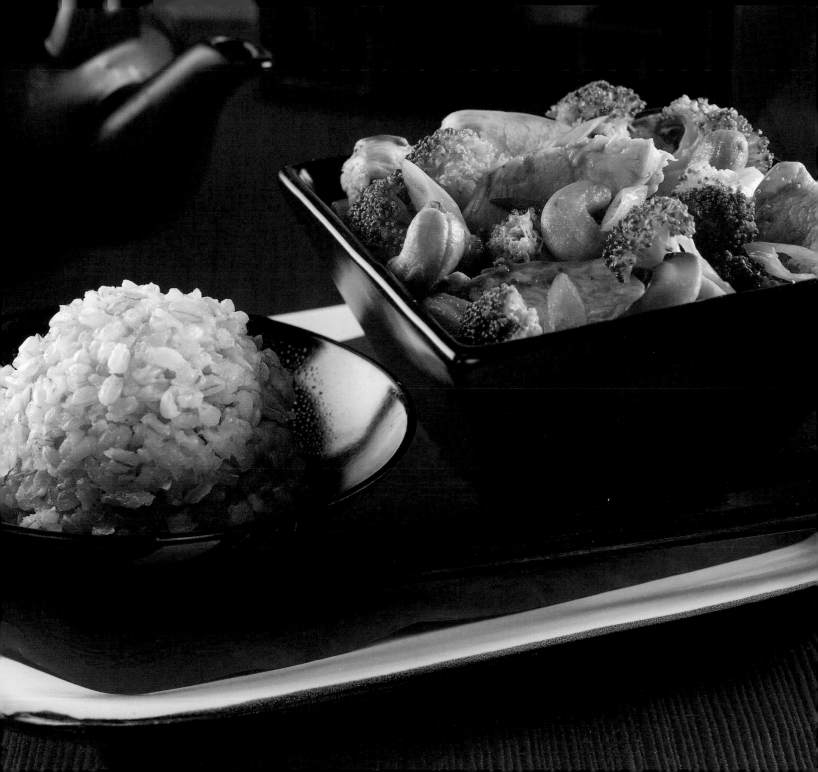

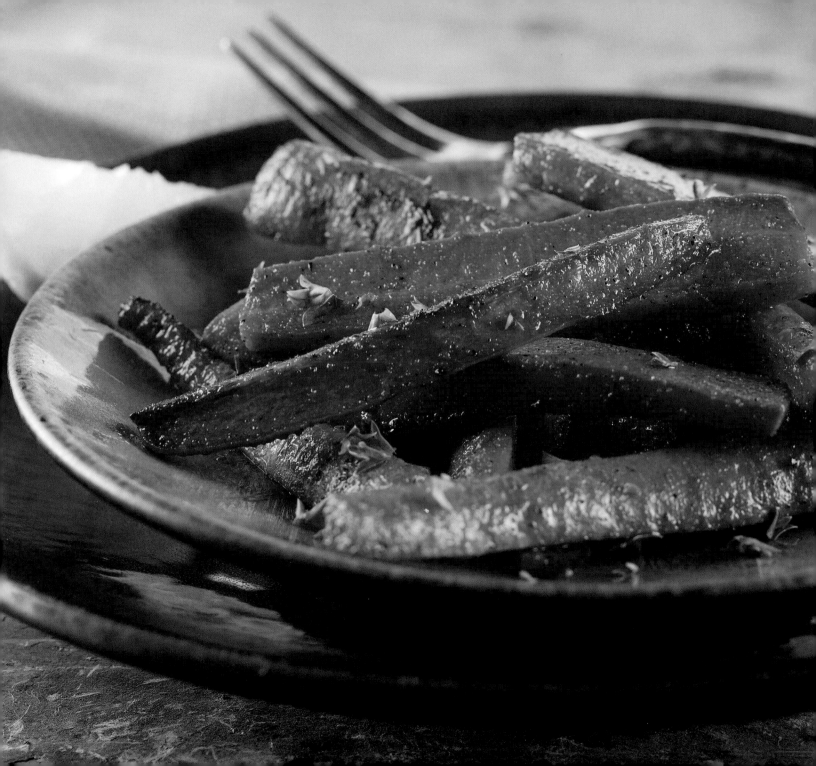

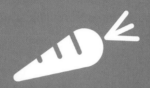

VEGETABLES

Since nutrient-rich vegetables are the cornerstone of a well-balanced diet—particularly when you're thinking about getting pregnant—this chapter answers the question of what to do with some of the most fertility-friendly veggies you'll find at the farmers' market or produce stand. All of these recipes are fast and easy enough to incorporate into a quick weeknight dinner. Some, like Spicy Green Beans, come together in well under ten minutes. Make Zucchini with Fennel and Tarragon when you're having chicken or fish. Or the next time your market has globe artichokes, try steaming them and dipping the leaves in a tasty red pepper aioli. These tasty sides will always find a place at the table.

Broccoli Purée with Parmesan Cheese

1 pound (454 grams)
broccoli florets, cut
into bite-size pieces*

1/3 cup (80 ml)
crème fraîche or sour cream*

1/4 cup (60 ml)
grated Parmesan cheese*

1/4 teaspoon (1.25 ml)
grated lemon zest

1/4 teaspoon
(1.25 ml) sea salt

1 to 2 tablespoons
(15 to 30 ml) milk

Freshly ground pepper

Broccoli is high in folate and antioxidants. It's enriched in this dish with whole-milk dairy, which may have benefits for fertility. This delicious, creamy purée makes a comforting, easy side dish for roast chicken or meats. Crème fraîche is a thick, silky cultured cream. If you can't find it, use sour cream instead.

Serves 4

1. Bring a large pot of lightly salted water to a boil. Add the broccoli and cook until very tender when pierced with a fork, 4 to 6 minutes. Drain well.

2. Transfer the broccoli to a food processor and add the crème fraîche, Parmesan, lemon zest, and salt. Whirl until smooth, adding milk as necessary to thin the purée.

3. Transfer to a bowl and season to taste with pepper and additional salt, if desired. Serve immediately.

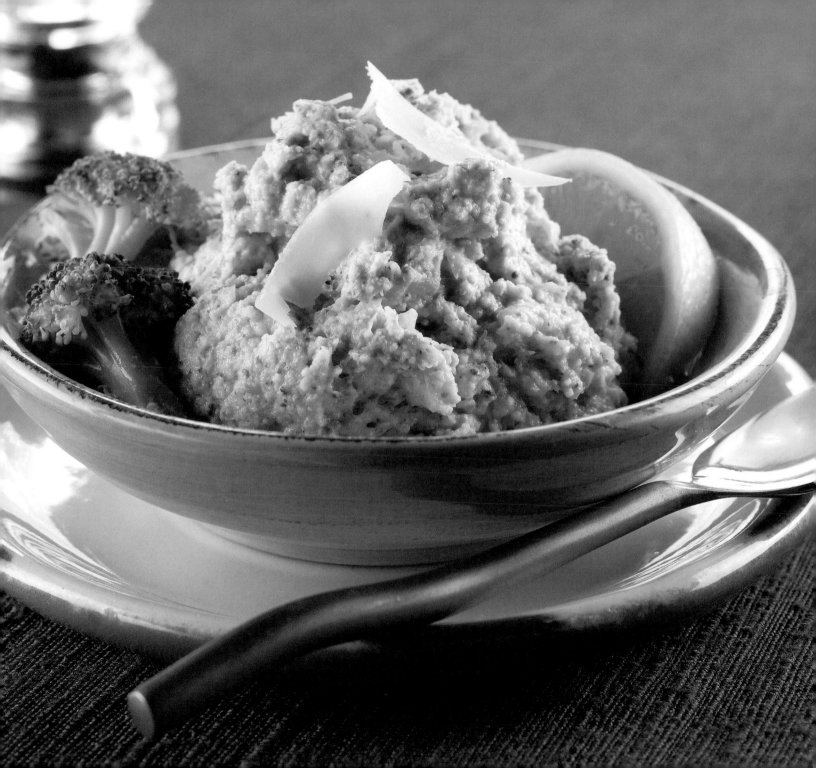

Zucchini with Fennel and Tarragon

3 tablespoons (45 ml) olive oil

½ cup (120 ml) leeks
(white and pale green
parts only), cut into
thin slices, rinsed well

1 fennel bulb, ends trimmed,
cut into thin slices*

½ teaspoon (2.5 ml) sea salt

Freshly ground black pepper

1 pound (454 grams)
zucchini, ends trimmed,
cut into 1-inch (25 mm) chunks*

1 tablespoon (15 ml)
chopped fresh tarragon leaves

Slowly cooked in olive oil and seasoned simply with sea salt and black pepper, this zucchini dish is a wonderful accompaniment to chicken or fish. It's easiest to wash the leeks after slicing them; just place them in a colander and rinse under running water until free of grit.

Serves 4

Heat the oil in a medium heavy-bottomed pot over medium heat. Add the leeks, fennel, salt, and a few grinds of pepper. Cook until the vegetables are soft but not brown, about 5 minutes. Stir in the zucchini and cover. Cook, stirring occasionally, until the zucchini is tender, about 15 minutes. Stir in the tarragon and season with additional salt and pepper to taste.

Roasted Asparagus with Hard-Cooked Egg Vinaigrette

This is a simple way to enjoy folate-rich asparagus, with a little extra iron and protein from the eggs. To cook the eggs, place them in a saucepan and cover with cold water. Bring the water to a boil over medium heat. Remove from the heat, cover, and let stand for 12 minutes. Carefully remove the eggs with a slotted spoon and place in a bowl of cold water until cool enough to peel.

Serves 4

1. Preheat the oven to 450°F (230°C).

2. In a shallow baking pan, drizzle the asparagus with 1 tablespoon (15 ml) of the olive oil and mix to coat. Sprinkle generously with salt and pepper. Roast until the asparagus is tender, about 10 minutes.

3. Stir together the lemon juice and the remaining olive oil in a bowl. Add the eggs, olives, capers, and parsley; mix gently to avoid mashing the yolks. Season to taste with salt and pepper.

4. Place the arugula on a serving plate. Arrange the asparagus on the arugula and spoon the egg vinaigrette over the asparagus. Serve warm or at room temperature.

---

1 1/2 pounds (681 grams) asparagus*

2 tablespoons (30 ml) extra-virgin olive oil, divided

Sea salt

Freshly ground pepper

1 tablespoon (15 ml) fresh lemon juice

2 hard-cooked eggs, coarsely chopped*

6 green olives, pitted and coarsely chopped

1/2 teaspoon (2.5 ml) capers, drained

1 tablespoon (15 ml) chopped fresh parsley

2 cups (480 ml) arugula or baby spinach leaves, washed*

Spicy Green Beans

12 ounces (336 grams)
green beans*

1 1/2 tablespoons
(22.5 ml) soy sauce

1 tablespoon (15 ml)
rice vinegar

1 teaspoon (5 ml) light or dark
brown sugar

1 tablespoon (15 ml) canola oil

1 shallot, peeled and minced

1 clove garlic, minced

1/2 teaspoon (2.5 ml)
Asian red chili paste or
1/4 teaspoon (1.25 ml)
crushed red pepper flakes

A light and spicy sauce coats these crisp stir-fried green beans, which are high in folate and antioxidants and are delicious with rice and simply broiled fish. If shallots are unavailable, you can substitute 2 tablespoons (30 ml) finely chopped red onion.

Serves 4

1. Trim the ends of the beans and cut them into 2-inch (51 mm) lengths. Bring a medium pot of water to a boil. Add the beans and cook just until crisp-tender, 3 to 4 minutes. Drain well. In a small bowl, stir together the soy sauce, rice vinegar, and sugar until the sugar is dissolved.

2. Heat the oil in a large frying pan over high heat. Add the shallot and garlic and cook until fragrant but not browned, about 45 seconds. Add the chili paste and the green beans and stir until the beans are heated through and well coated, about 2 minutes. Add the soy sauce mixture and cook until the liquid reduces slightly and the beans are tender, about 1 minute longer.

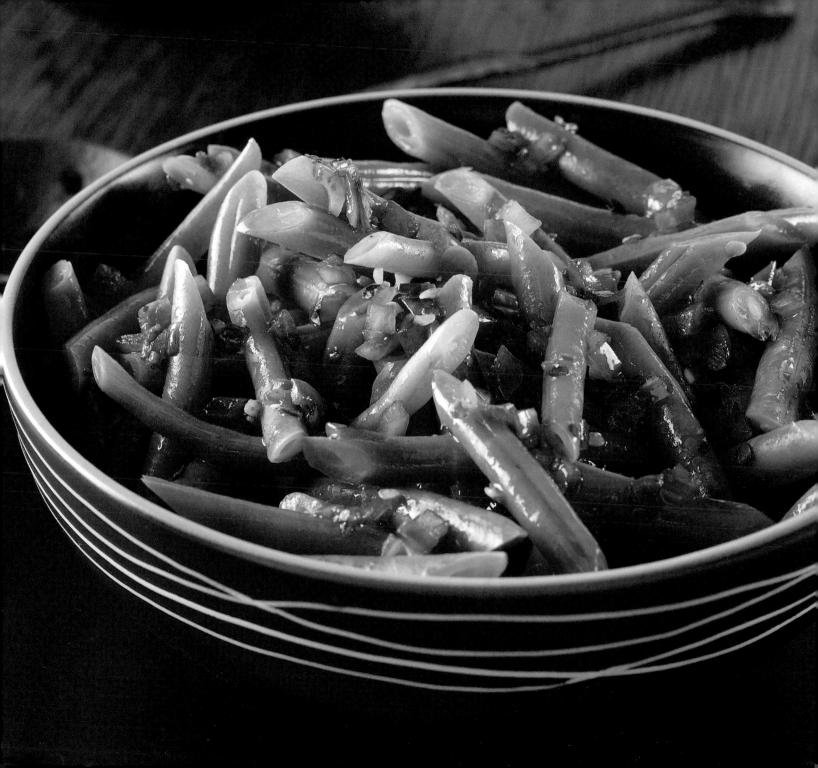

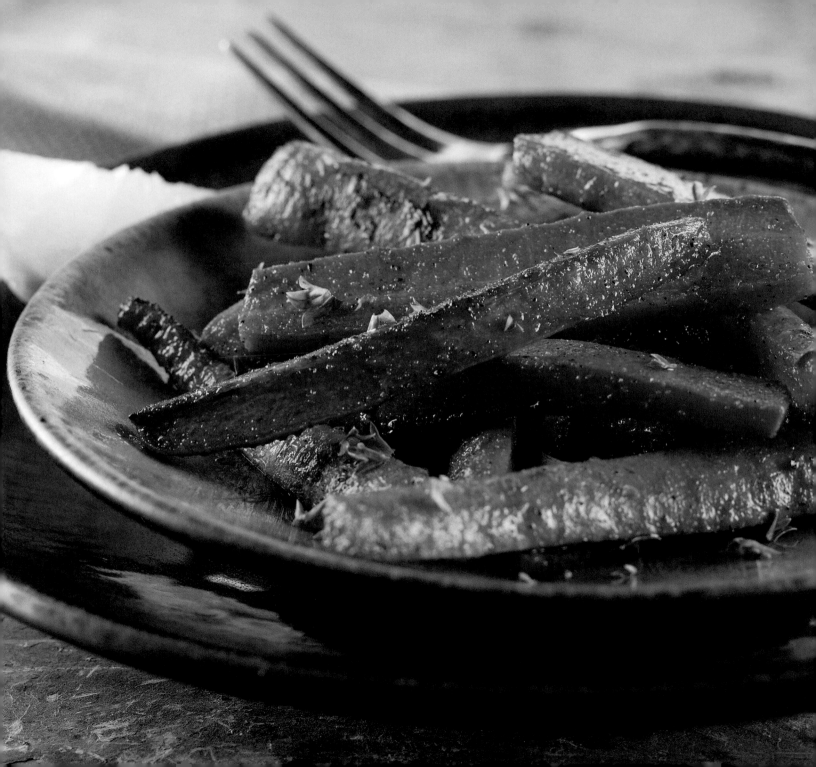

Carmelized Carrots

Low-calorie and sweet, carrots are a great fresh vegetable side dish. Small, slender baby carrots are especially pretty in this dish. Just trim the top ends and roast them whole.

Serves 4

1. Preheat the oven to 400°F (200°C).

2. Scrub the carrots and trim the top ends. Cut each carrot in half crosswise to make pieces about 3 to 4 inches (76 to 102 mm) long, and then cut them in half again lengthwise. Cut the pieces into sticks that are 1/4-inch (6 mm) thick. Place in a large roasting pan and add the oil, salt, cumin, paprika, and a few grinds of pepper. Mix well to coat.

3. Bake, stirring after 10 minutes, until the carrots are tender and beginning to caramelize around the edges, 18 to 25 minutes total. Remove from the oven and mix with the parsley and lemon juice.

1 1/2 pounds (681 grams) carrots*

1 1/2 tablespoons (22.5 ml) olive oil

1/2 teaspoon (2.5 ml) sea salt

1/2 teaspoon (2.5 ml) ground cumin

1/4 teaspoon (1.25 ml) smoked paprika

Freshly ground pepper

1 1/2 tablespoons (22.5 ml) chopped fresh parsley

1 teaspoon (5 ml) fresh lemon juice

Roasted Beets with Orange Vinaigrette

2½ pounds (about 1.1 kilograms, including tops) small beets*

2 teaspoons (10 ml) fresh orange juice*

3 tablespoons (45 ml) white wine vinegar

2 tablespoons (30 ml) olive oil

2 tablespoons (30 ml) minced red onion or shallots

¼ teaspoon (1.25 ml) salt

Freshly ground pepper

Fresh beets are a sweet treat, particularly in spring and fall, when you can buy them in colorful bundles at the market. They are also a source of iron and the important nutrient *folate*. Roasted until tender and dressed simply with a light vinaigrette, they make an easy, versatile side dish.

Serves 4

1. Preheat the oven to 375°F (190°C).

2. Rinse the beets well and trim off the greens, leaving 1 inch (25 mm) of each stem. Place the beets in a baking pan and fill the pan with about ½ inch (12.7 mm) water. Cover tightly with foil and bake until tender when pierced, 30 to 45 minutes. When cool enough to handle, peel and cut into ½-inch (12.7 mm) wedges.

3. Meanwhile, in a bowl, combine the orange juice, vinegar, oil, onion, salt, and pepper to taste. Add the warm beets and stir to coat. Serve warm or at room temperature.

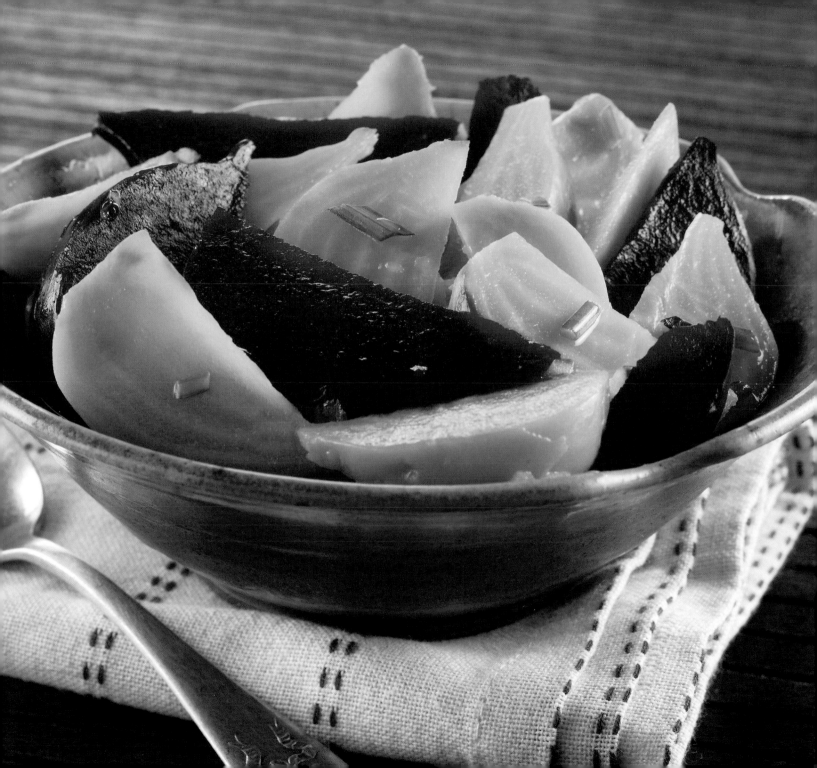

Slow-Roasted Tomatoes

2 tablespoons (30 ml) olive oil, plus more for the pan

3 pounds (1.4 kilograms) small tomatoes, such as Roma*

2 tablespoons (30 ml) balsamic vinegar

1 clove garlic, minced

1/2 teaspoon (2.5 ml) dried oregano

Sea salt

Freshly ground pepper

Sweet and tender, roasted lycopene-rich tomatoes make a great side dish at brunch or dinner, and they're a nice addition to sandwiches, soups, or cooked pasta. Roma or medium-sized round tomatoes work best for this recipe.

Serves 4

1. Preheat the oven to 300°F (150°C). Lightly oil a roasting pan or a large baking dish. Cut the tomatoes in half lengthwise and place them cut side up in the prepared pan.

2. In a small bowl, mix oil, vinegar, garlic, and oregano. Spoon the mixture evenly over the tomatoes and sprinkle the tomatoes lightly with salt and pepper. Bake until the tomatoes are soft and wrinkled, 45 minutes to 1 hour.

FERTILITY FACT:

Tomatoes contain lycopene, an important fertility ingredient for men. Lycopene is actually better absorbed by the body once tomatoes are processed into soup, juice, or sauce.

Steamed Artichokes with Red Pepper Aioli

Artichokes may look like they're tough to tackle, but they're actually very easy to prepare and they're a great source of folate. Feel free to substitute reduced-fat mayonnaise in this tangy dip, if you prefer.

Serves 4

1. In a blender or food processor, combine the mayonnaise, red peppers, garlic, 1 tablespoon (15 ml) of the lemon juice, and the paprika. Whirl until smooth. Season to taste with salt and pepper and spoon into a small bowl for dipping and set aside.

2. Bring a pot of salted water to a boil and add the remaining lemon juice. Trim the artichoke stem ends. Remove the tough outer leaves around the base of the artichokes, and use a sharp paring knife to remove the fibrous peel from the stems. With a large, sharp knife, cut about 1 inch (25 mm) off the top of each artichoke. Boil the artichokes until the base is tender when pierced with a knife, 20 to 25 minutes. Remove from the water with tongs and set aside, upside down, until cool enough to handle.

3. Serve with the red pepper aioli for dipping.

1/3 cup (80 ml) prepared mayonnaise

*1/3 cup (80 ml) coarsely chopped jarred roasted red peppers**

1 clove garlic, peeled and crushed

5 tablespoons (75 ml) fresh lemon juice, divided

1/2 teaspoon (2.5 ml) paprika

Sea salt

Freshly ground pepper

*4 large artichokes (about 1 pound or 454 grams each)**

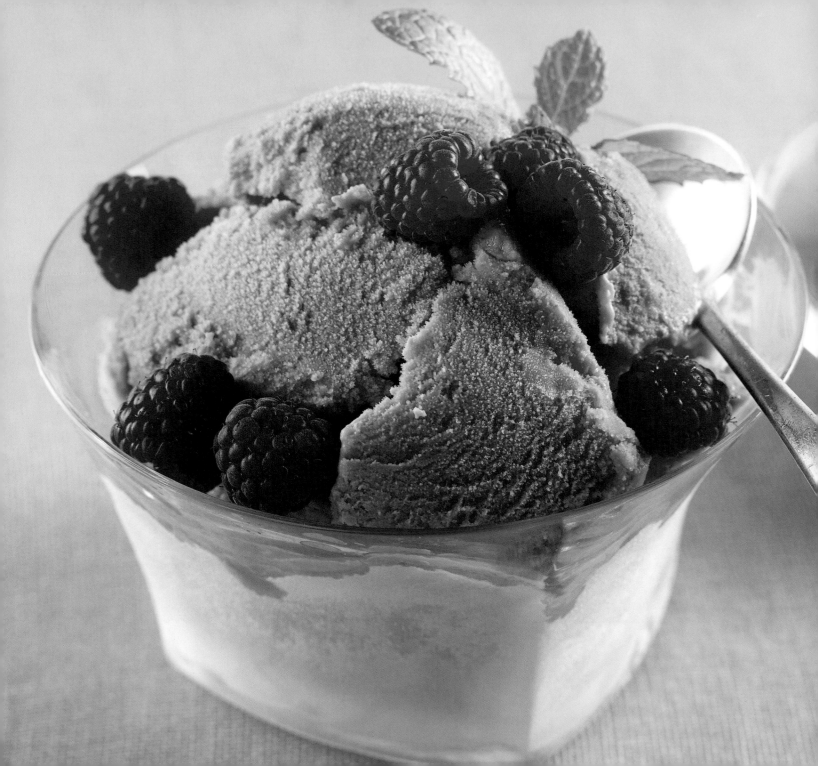

DESSERTS

What could be sweeter than indulging in a delicious dessert—and knowing you're getting nutrients you need to get your body ready for pregnancy? In this chapter, you'll be able to have your cookies and eat them, too. Polenta Biscotti are studded with iron and fiber-rich dried fruit, as well as omega-3-rich pistachios, and make a sweet bite after dinner. There are lots of opportunities to get a serving of fertility-friendly whole-milk dairy, including Creamy Chocolate Pudding and tangy Raspberry Frozen Yogurt. And desserts like Chocolate Cheesecake Brownies, made with omega-3-rich canola oil, are likely to be favorites for years to come. Of course, moderation is the key for a healthy diet, but it's nice to know that when you do decide to indulge, you're getting a wholesome treat made with nutritious ingredients.

Broiled Peaches with Vanilla Sour Cream

½ cup (120 ml) sour cream*

3 tablespoons (45 ml) sugar, divided

1 teaspoon (5 ml) grated orange zest

¼ teaspoon (1.25 ml) vanilla extract

2 firm-ripe freestone peaches*

A ripe, fresh peach is a nearly perfect dessert all by itself, but heating peaches under the broiler for a few minutes concentrates their flavor and sweetness. Topped with lightly sweetened sour cream, they're irresistible, and special enough for a dinner party. If you have any leftover Polenta Biscotti (page 137), they make a nice accompaniment.

Serves 2

1. In a small bowl, whisk together the sour cream, 2 tablespoons (30 ml) of the sugar, the orange zest, and vanilla until smooth.

2. Preheat the broiler. Line a baking sheet with foil.

3. Cut the peaches in half and remove the pits. Cut a thin slice off the rounded side of each peach half so that it sits flat, cut-side up. Place on the baking sheet. Sprinkle the cut sides of the peaches evenly with the remaining sugar.

4. Broil 4 to 5 inches from the heat until the sugar is melted and bubbling and the peaches are tender, 6 to 8 minutes.

5. Serve with the sweetened sour cream.

Optional: To add omega-3s, sprinkle with 1 tablespoon (15 ml) chopped pistachios.

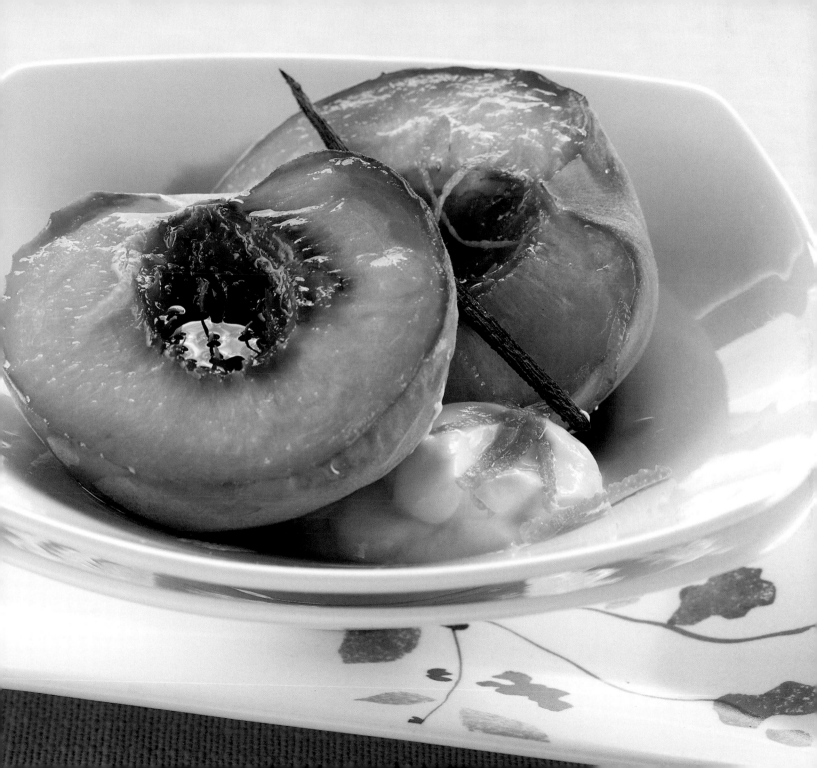

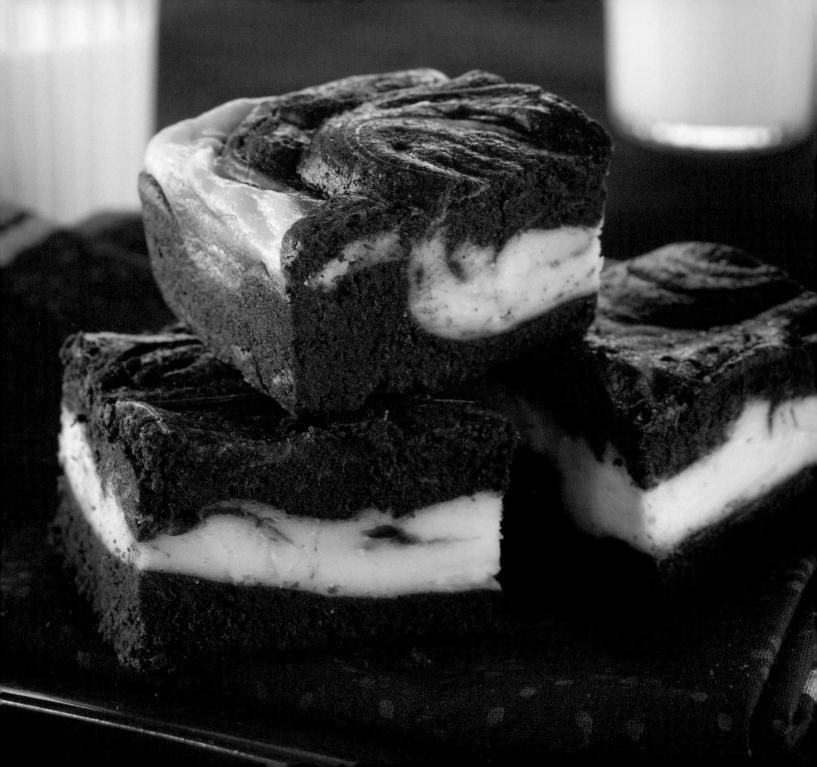

Chocolate Cheesecake Brownies

If you're a brownie fan, these ultra-chocolaty brownies with a cream cheese swirl are likely to become your new favorites. If you don't have time to bring the cream cheese to room temperature, you can soften it (unwrapped on a plate) in the microwave for a few seconds. Omega-3-rich canola oil replaces the usual butter in these rich brownies, and dark chocolate is high in antioxidants.

Makes 16 brownies

1. Preheat the oven to 325°F (160°C). Lightly oil an 8-inch-square (203-mm-square) baking pan and lightly dust the bottom with flour.

2. Place the chocolate in a heatproof bowl and set over a pan of barely simmering water. Stir the chocolate frequently until melted and smooth. Remove the bowl from the pan and whisk in the oil, 3/4 cup (178 ml) of the sugar, and the vanilla. Whisk in 3 eggs, one at a time, beating well after each addition. Stir in the flour and salt just until blended.

3. In another bowl, with a wooden spoon or a mixer, beat the cream cheese with the remaining sugar until smooth. Beat in the remaining egg until smoothly incorporated.

4. Spread about two-thirds of the chocolate mixture in the prepared pan. Spoon the cream cheese mixture evenly over the chocolate. Spoon the remaining chocolate mixture on top, partially but not completely covering the cheese mixture. Drag a butter knife through the batter to swirl the mixtures slightly.

5. Bake until the edges are set and a wooden skewer inserted into the center comes out with moist crumbs attached, 35 to 40 minutes. Let cool in pan on a rack for at least 20 minutes (brownies will firm up as they cool), then cut into 16 squares.

6 ounces (170 grams) bittersweet chocolate, finely chopped*

1/2 cup (120 ml) canola oil, plus more for the pan*

1 cup (240 ml) sugar, divided

1 1/2 teaspoons (7.5 ml) vanilla extract

4 large eggs, divided

3/4 cup (178 ml) all-purpose flour, plus more for the pan

1/4 teaspoon (1.25 ml) salt

8 ounces (227 grams) cream cheese, at room temperature*

Chocolate Chip Cookies with Walnuts and Cherries

1/2 cup (120 ml) butter at room temperature

1 cup (240 ml) light brown sugar

2 large eggs

1 teaspoon (5 ml) vanilla extract

1 cup (240 ml) all-purpose flour

3/4 cup (178 ml) whole-wheat flour*

1/4 cup (60 ml) wheat germ*

2 tablespoons (30 ml) ground flaxseed*

1 teaspoon (5 ml) baking soda

1/2 teaspoon (2.5 ml) salt

1 cup (240 ml) finely chopped bittersweet chocolate*

1/2 cup (120 ml) chopped walnuts*

1/2 cup (120 ml) dried sour cherries*

Chocolate chip cookies are everybody's favorite. This scrumptious version is fortified with dried cherries for extra flavor and fiber, plus ground flaxseed, wheat germ, and antioxidant- and fiber-rich walnuts and dark chocolate. Look for ground flaxseed at natural foods stores.

Makes about 36 cookies

1. Preheat the oven to 375°F (190°C). Line two baking sheets with parchment paper.

2. In a bowl, with a mixer on medium speed, beat the butter and brown sugar until smooth and creamy. Beat in the eggs and vanilla until well blended, scraping down the sides of the bowl as needed.

3. In another bowl, mix the flours, wheat germ, flaxseed, baking soda, and salt. Stir or beat into the butter mixture until well incorporated. Stir in the chocolate, nuts, and cherries.

4. Drop dough in heaping tablespoon-size portions, about 2 inches (51 mm) apart, onto the baking sheets. Bake until the cookies are lightly browned at the edges and feel firm to the touch, 8 to 11 minutes. If baking more than one pan at a time, switch pan positions halfway through baking. With a wide spatula, transfer the cookies to racks to cool.

Three-Berry Oatmeal Crumble

Make this juicy crumble at the height of summer, when the antioxidant-rich fruit is ripe, plentiful, and inexpensive. Berries vary in sweetness, and blackberries in particular can sometimes be quite sour. Taste the berries first; if they are very tart, you might want to add the additional tablespoon of sugar.

Serves 8

1. To make the topping: In a bowl, mix the oats, flour, brown sugar, and salt. Rub the butter into the dry ingredients with your fingers or a fork until the mixture forms coarse, uniform crumbs. Stir in the almonds. Preheat the oven to 375°F (190°C).

2. To make the filling: In a large bowl, stir together the sugar and cornstarch. Add the berries and toss to coat. Pour the berries into a shallow 2¹/₂- to 3-quart baking dish. Sprinkle the top evenly with the topping.

3. Bake until the topping is golden brown and the juices are bubbling, 35 to 40 minutes. Let stand for at least 10 minutes before serving.

Oatmeal-Almond Topping:

1¹/₄ cups (300 ml) rolled oats*

¹/₂ cup (120 ml) whole-wheat flour*

¹/₂ cup (120 ml) packed light brown sugar

¹/₄ teaspoon (1.25 ml) salt

6 tablespoons (90 ml) butter, cut into chunks

¹/₂ cup (120 ml) chopped almonds*

Filling

3 to 4 tablespoons (45 to 60 ml) granulated sugar

1 tablespoon (15 ml) cornstarch

6 cups (1.4 liters) fresh berries, such as raspberries, blackberries, or blueberries*

FERTILITY FACT:
Complex carbohydrates like whole grains (oatmeal is one example) and fruit not only supply key nutrients but can actually improve ovulation and increase your chances of getting pregnant.

Pumpkin Gingerbread

1/2 cup (120 ml) canola oil, plus more for the pan*

3/4 cup (178 ml) light brown sugar, packed

3 eggs

1 cup (240 ml) canned pumpkin purée*

1/2 cup (120 ml) dark molasses*

2 cups (480 ml) whole-wheat flour*

1 teaspoon (5 ml) baking powder

1/2 teaspoon (2.5 ml) baking soda

1/2 teaspoon (2.5 ml) salt

1/2 teaspoon (2.5 ml) ground nutmeg*

1/2 teaspoon (2.5 ml) ground cinnamon*

1/2 teaspoon (2.5 ml) ground ginger*

1/4 teaspoon (1.25 ml) ground cloves*

1/4 cup (60 ml) whole milk*

Powdered sugar for garnishing

This spice cake gets its golden color and moist texture from pumpkin purée, which also contributes vitamins and antioxidants. Tangy molasses adds sweetness, plus iron, calcium, and folate. It's a lovely, not-too-sweet Thanksgiving dessert. It's also a delicious snack cake any time of the year. Serve with a dollop of whipped cream.

Serves 8 to 9

1. Preheat the oven to 350°F (180°C). Lightly oil an 8-inch-square (203-mm-square) baking pan.

2. In a large bowl, whisk together the oil, brown sugar, eggs, pumpkin, and molasses.

3. In a small bowl, stir together the flour, baking powder, baking soda, salt, nutmeg, cinnamon, ginger, and cloves. Fold gently into the pumpkin mixture. Stir in the milk just until blended.

4. Pour into the prepared pan and bake until a wooden skewer inserted into the center comes out clean, 40 to 45 minutes. Let cool in the pan for 15 minutes, then cut into squares and serve warm, or allow it to cool completely. Sprinkle the top with powdered sugar before serving.

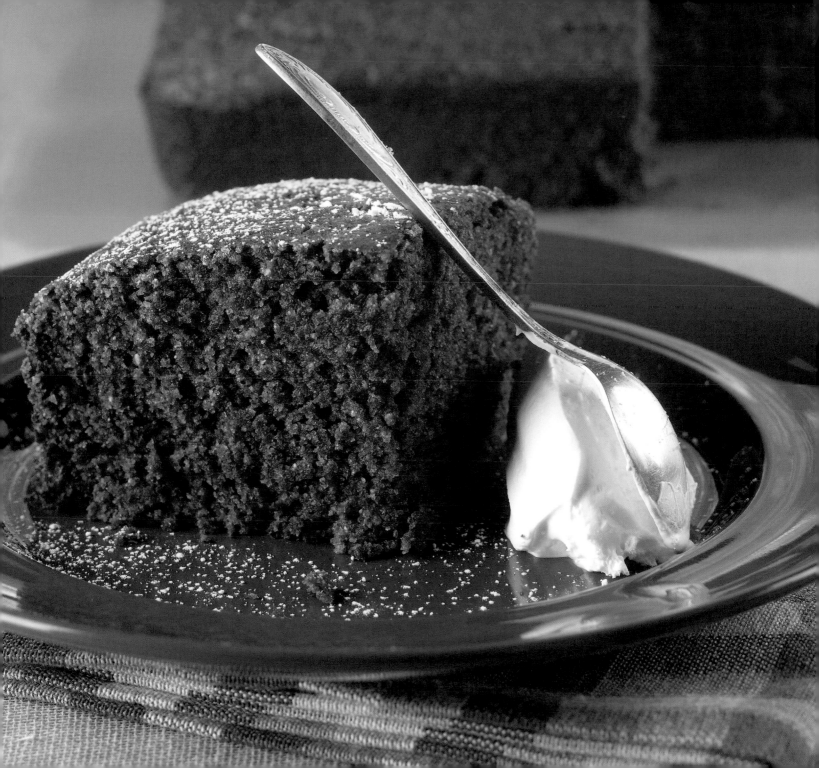

Creamy Chocolate Pudding

2 cups (480 ml) whole milk *

2 large egg yolks

1/4 cup (60 ml) sugar

2 tablespoons (30 ml) cornstarch

1/8 teaspoon (.5 ml) salt

4 ounces (113 grams)
bittersweet chocolate,
finely chopped *

1/2 teaspoon (2.5 ml)
vanilla extract

This silky, rich treat is made with calcium-rich whole milk, and gets anti-oxidants from dark chocolate. It's the ultimate comfort food, perfect for a cozy night in front of the TV or an informal gathering of friends. Use a large sharp knife to finely chop the chocolate.

Serves 4 to 6

1. In a medium saucepan, whisk together the milk and egg yolks. In a small bowl, stir together the sugar, cornstarch, and salt. Whisk the sugar mixture into milk mixture.

2. Bring the mixture to a simmer over medium heat, stirring constantly with a flexible spatula or a wooden spoon, 5 to 6 minutes. When the mixture begins to bubble around the edges, cook it gently for 1 minute, stirring constantly, and then remove from the heat. Whisk in the chocolate until melted and smooth, followed by the vanilla.

3. Spoon the pudding into individual bowls, dessert glasses, or a large serving bowl and place a piece of wax paper directly on the surface of the pudding to prevent a skin from forming. Chill until cold, about 2 hours.

FERTILITY FACT:
It may be difficult to think of creamy ice cream, yogurt, or pudding as health foods, but when you're trying to conceive, a serving or two a day of full-fat dairy (rather than nonfat) seems to protect against infertility. The estrogen and progesterone in milk are attached to the fat, as opposed to other hormones in dairy products that are not conducive to conception but are left behind when the fat is skimmed off.

Baked Apples with Dates and Walnuts

Fill the kitchen with a wonderful scent as you bake this warm, low-calorie fall dessert. Any leftover apples are wonderful for breakfast with plain or vanilla yogurt.

Serves 4

1. Preheat the oven to 350°F (180°C). Lightly butter an 8- or 9-inch (203- or 209-mm) baking dish.

2. Cut a thin slice off the stem end of each apple and use a melon baller to remove the core and a little bit from the center to make a cavity for the filling, taking care to leave the bottom of the apple intact.

3. In a bowl, stir together the walnuts, dates, cracker crumbs, maple syrup, lemon juice, cinnamon, and salt until well blended. Spoon the mixture into the apple centers. Place the apples in prepared baking dish and pour the cider into the bottom of the dish. Dot the exposed filling on the top of each apple with two small pieces of butter. Cover the dish tightly with foil and bake until the apples are tender when pierced, 50 to 60 minutes.

4. Transfer the apples to plates and spoon the juice over the apples.

*4 large sweet apples, such as Gala**

*1/2 cup (120 ml) finely chopped walnuts**

1/3 cup (80 ml) pitted and finely chopped dates

1/3 cup (80 ml) coarsely crumbled graham crackers

1 tablespoon (15 ml) maple syrup

Juice of half a lemon

*1/2 teaspoon (2.5 ml) ground cinnamon**

Pinch of salt

1/2 cup (120 ml) apple cider or juice

1 tablespoon (15 ml) butter, cut into 8 small pieces, plus more for preparing pan

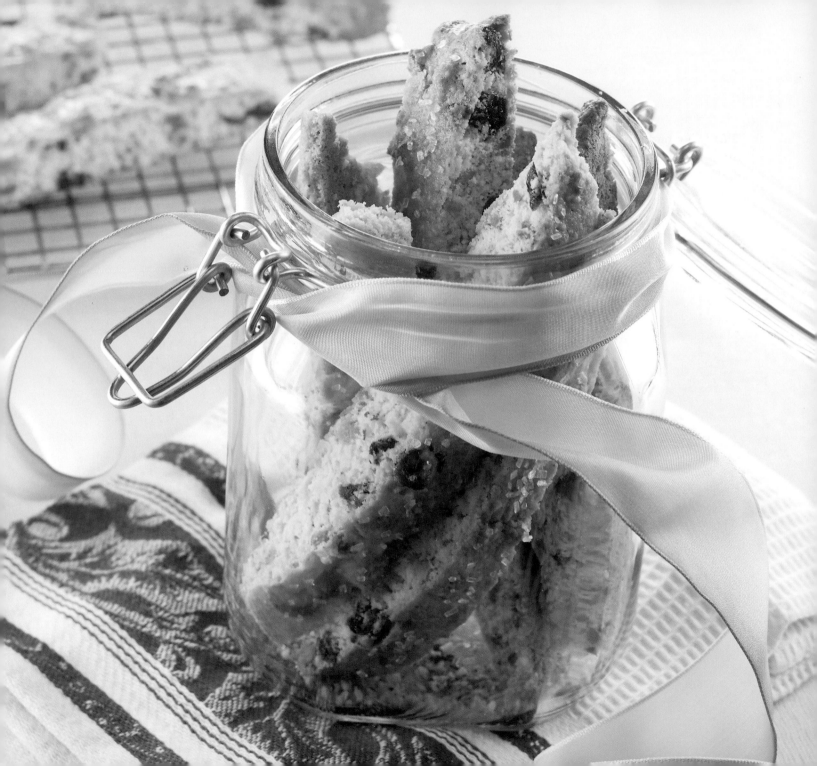

Polenta Biscotti with Pistachios and Dried Fruit

This is a wonderful little dunking cookie, studded with iron- and fiber-rich dried fruit and pistachios. It's even more sublime when dipped in melted dark chocolate! The stone-ground cornmeal gives the cookies a crumbly, slightly sandy texture.

Makes about 36 cookies

1. Preheat the oven to 375°F (190°C). Line two baking sheets with parchment paper.

2. In a medium bowl, stir together the flour, cornmeal, baking powder, and salt.

3. In a large bowl, with a mixer on high speed or a wooden spoon, beat the butter and sugar until smooth and well blended. Beat in the eggs, one at a time, beating well after each addition. Beat in the vanilla and lemon zest. Stir the flour mixture into the butter mixture until just incorporated. Stir in the pistachios and dried fruit.

4. Spoon the dough (it will be sticky) onto the prepared baking sheets in four even strips, each about 2 inches (51 mm) wide and 12 inches (305 mm) long.

5. Bake until the strips are firm to the touch and light golden brown, switching pan positions after 10 minutes, baking 18 to 20 minutes in total. Remove from the oven and let stand until cool enough to handle, about 15 minutes. Reduce the oven temperature to 300°F (150°C).

6. With a large serrated knife, carefully slice the strips on the diagonal into 3/4-inch-wide (19-mm-wide) cookies. Spread the slices out on the baking pan, return to the oven, and bake until lightly golden brown, about 15 minutes longer. Let cool completely and transfer to an airtight container to store.

1 2/3 cups (390 ml) all-purpose flour

3/4 cup (180 ml) stone-ground cornmeal (polenta)*

2 teaspoons (10 ml) baking powder

1/2 teaspoon (2.5 ml) salt

1/2 cup (120 ml) unsalted butter at room temperature

1 cup (240 ml) sugar

3 large eggs

1 teaspoon (5 ml) vanilla extract

Grated zest of 1 lemon

3/4 cup (178 ml) coarsely chopped pistachios*

1/3 cup (80 ml) dried cranberries*

1/3 cup (80 ml) diced dried apricots*

1/3 cup (80 ml) currants or golden raisins*

Raspberry Frozen Yogurt

2 cups (8 ounces or 227 grams) fresh raspberries*

1 cup (240 ml) sugar, divided

3 cups (720 ml) plain whole-milk yogurt*

1 tablespoon (15 ml) vanilla extract

1 teaspoon (5 ml) fresh lemon juice

Raspberries are sweet packages of vitamins and antioxidants. When they are at the peak of their sweetness, this tangy frozen treat, made with calcium-rich whole-milk yogurt, is the dessert to make. The frozen yogurt will have the best texture the first day or two after you make it.

Serves 6 to 8; makes about 1 quart

1. In a food processor, whirl the raspberries with 1/4 cup (60 ml) of the sugar. Pour through a strainer into a large bowl, pressing on the solids with a spoon to extract as much juice as possible; discard the seeds.

2. Whisk in the yogurt, vanilla, lemon juice, and the remaining sugar until the sugar is dissolved.

3. Freeze in an ice-cream maker according to the manufacturer's instructions.

4. Serve immediately, or transfer to an airtight container and freeze until firm, about 4 hours.

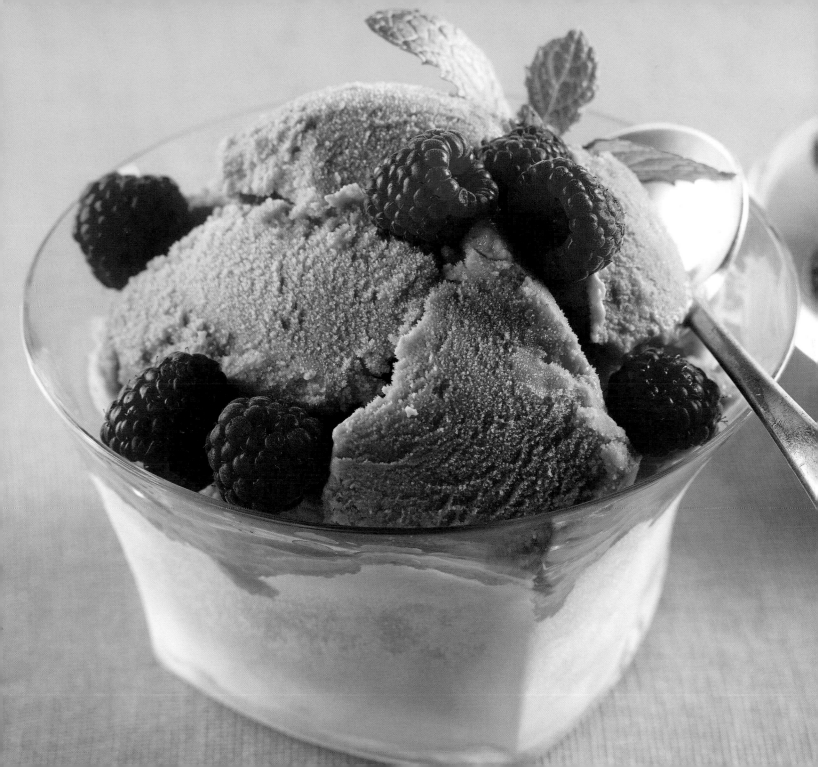

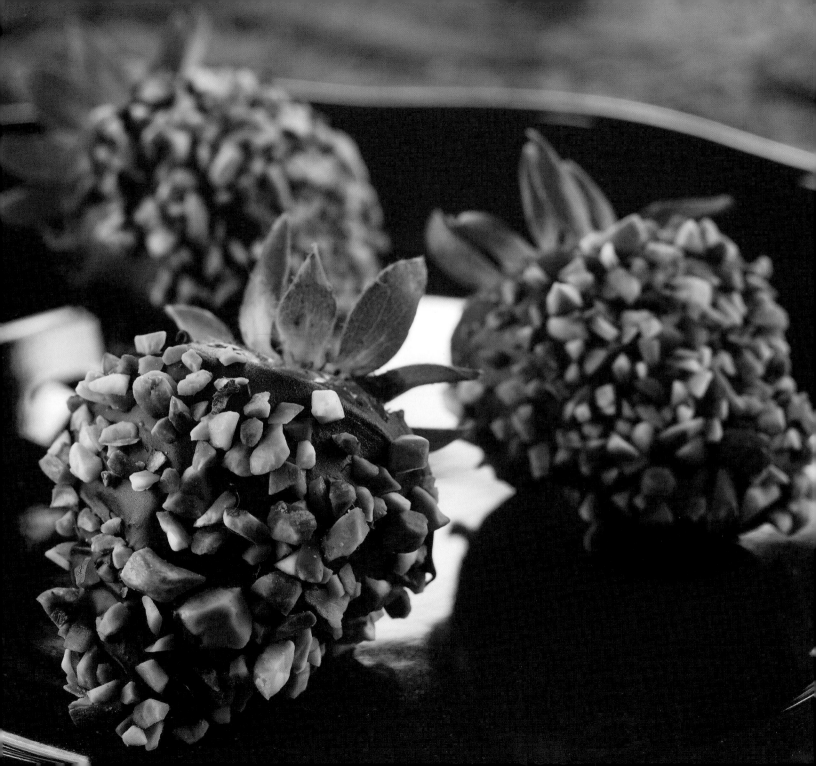

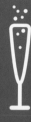

RECIPES FOR ROMANCE

Food and romance go hand in hand. Cooking a special meal together to eat by candlelight can ignite the mood *and* support fertility. You'll bask in the glow of knowing that the filet mignon you're making is an excellent source of zinc for healthy sperm production. In this chapter, you'll also find a menu for a special, cozy breakfast in bed to celebrate a weekend of baby making, and some recipes for tasty "mocktails" that have all the fun without the alcohol.

Poached Eggs with Red Pepper–Walnut Purée

Red Pepper–Walnut Purée

One 8-ounce (227 gram) jar roasted red bell peppers, drained*

1/4 cup (60ml) walnut pieces, lightly toasted*

1 clove garlic

3 tablespoons (45 ml) olive oil

2 teaspoons (10 ml) balsamic or red wine vinegar

1/2 teaspoon (2.5 ml) smoked paprika

1/4 teaspoon (1.25 ml) ground cumin

1/4 teaspoon (1.25 ml) salt

Poached Eggs

8 slender asparagus spears*

2 whole-wheat English muffins*

4 large eggs

Sea salt

Freshly ground pepper

4 slices (1/2 ounce or 14 grams each) Havarti cheese*

Share this dish to celebrate a leisurely morning in bed. Eggs contain iron, asparagus is a great source of folate, and the savory pureé of walnuts and peppers is full of omega-3s and antioxidants. Havarti cheese is often sold sliced in the grocery's deli section. If you can't find it, opt for any good melting cheese like white Cheddar, provolone, or Monterey Jack.

This recipe makes more Red Pepper–Walnut Pureé than you'll need for this dish. The extra will keep in the refrigerator for a week, and is great on sandwiches, crackers, or pasta.

Serves 2

1. To make the Red Pepper–Walnut Purée: In a blender, whirl all of the ingredients until smooth. Makes about 1 cup (240 ml).

2. To make the poached eggs: Trim the bottom portion of the asparagus spears to get spears that are about 4 inches (102 mm) long. Bring a deep frying pan of lightly salted water to a boil. Add the asparagus and boil for 2 minutes, until just tender. Remove from the water with a slotted spoon and drain well. Keep the water in the pan to cook the eggs.

3. Preheat the broiler. Cut the muffins in half horizontally and place on a baking sheet. Spread the cut side of each muffin half with red pepper purée.

4. Adjust the heat under the frying pan to maintain a simmer. Crack the eggs, 1 at a time, into a measuring cup, then gently slide into the water. Cook for 3 minutes or until eggs are softly set.

5. Remove the eggs from the water with a slotted spoon and place 1 egg on each muffin half. Sprinkle with salt and pepper. Arrange two asparagus spears over each egg in an X pattern. Top with a slice of cheese and place under the broiler just to melt the cheese (watch carefully to prevent burning), about 1 minute. Serve immediately with additional red pepper purée on the side.

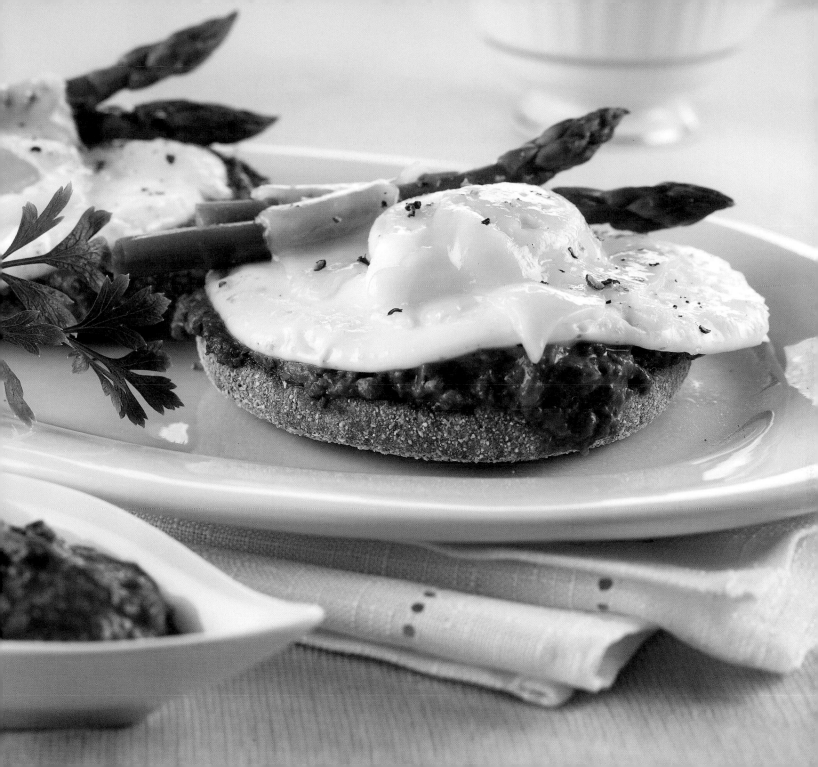

Tangerine Mimosas

1 tablespoon (15 ml) honey

1 1/2 teaspoons (7.5 ml) fresh lime juice

1 cup (240 ml) fresh tangerine juice*

1 cup (240 ml) sparkling water or club soda

Breakfast in bed calls for a pretty sparkling drink in a champagne flute. Get all of the folate-rich juice without the alcohol in this version of mimosas. (Note: This nonalcoholic drink, and the others in this chapter, are not necessarily high in fertility-boosting nutrients, but are presented as a healthy alternative to drinking alcohol when trying to conceive.)

Serves 2

In a small bowl, stir together the honey and lime juice. Pour the tangerine juice into a small pitcher and stir in the honey mixture until dissolved. Add the sparkling water and pour into glasses.

FERTILITY FACT:

Try to quit or reduce your soft drink habit when you're trying to conceive. The sugar and caffeine in these drinks can negatively affect blood sugar and insulin levels, a concern especially for women with PCOS, a common fertility-spoiler. Switch to sugar-free sodas if you must, or find healthy beverage alternatives.

Strawberry-Grapefruit Compote

Ruby grapefruit, a source of lycopene, and red strawberries make a beautiful morning compote.

Serves 2

1. With a sharp knife, cut off and discard the ends from the grapefruit. Carefully trim away the peel and outer membrane, following the curve of the fruit. With your fingers or the knife, gently remove the segments from the inner membranes and place in a shallow bowl; discard the membranes.

2. Gently stir in the strawberries, sugar, vanilla, and mint. Cover and chill for at least 30 minutes.

1 large or 2 small ruby grapefruits (about 1 pound or 454 grams total)

1 cup (240 ml) fresh strawberries, cut into slices*

1 tablespoon (15 ml) light brown sugar

1/2 teaspoon (2.5 ml) vanilla

2 or 3 thinly slivered fresh mint leaves

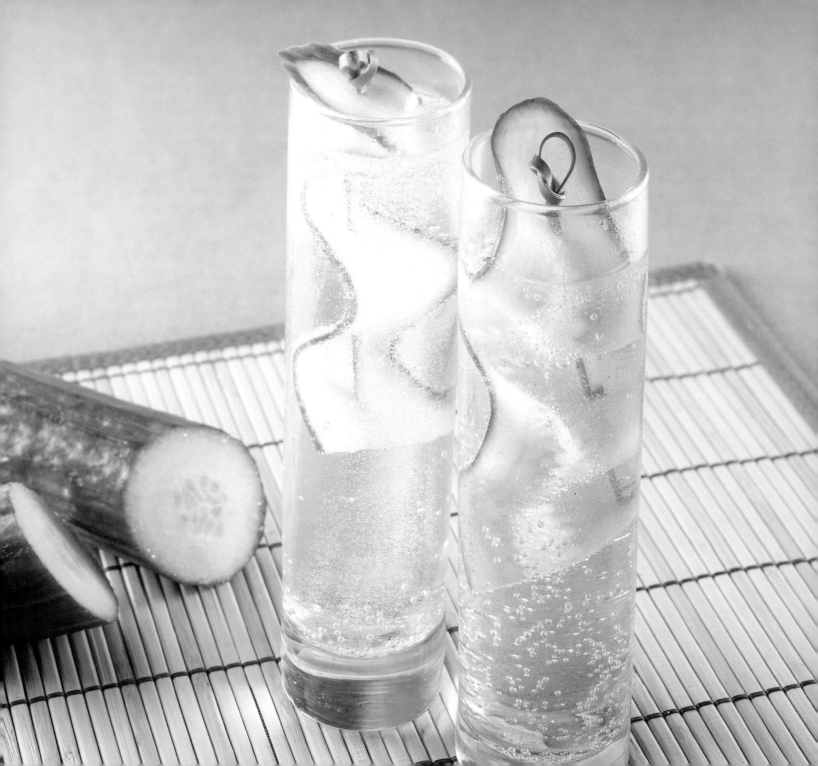

Cucumber Tonic

Part spa water, part classy cocktail: sip this refreshing beverage from a highball glass, over ice if you like. Use a thin-skinned English or Persian cucumber if you can; otherwise, peel the thick waxy skin from a regular cucumber.

Serves 2

Place 3 cucumber slices in each of two glasses. To each glass, add 1 cup (240 ml) tonic water and 1/2 teaspoon (2.5 ml) lime juice. Add ice if desired. Make a small cut in the remaining two cucumber slices and place one over the rim of each glass.

8 thin cucumber slices

2 cups (480 ml) tonic water

1 teaspoon (5 ml) fresh lime juice

Ice cubes (optional)

Pomegranate Spritzer

*1/2 cup (120 ml) pomegranate juice**

1 1/2 cups (360 ml) club soda or sparkling water

1 teaspoon (5 ml) fresh lime juice

2 strips lime peel

Fresh pomegranate juice is increasingly available in the refrigerated sections of many supermarkets. Serve these tangy pink drinks in martini glasses for a nonalcoholic night in.

Serves 2

In each of two martini glasses, combine 1/4 cup (60 ml) pomegranate juice, 3/4 cup (178 ml) club soda, and 1/2 teaspoon (2.5 ml) lime juice. Garnish each glass with a strip of lime peel and serve immediately.

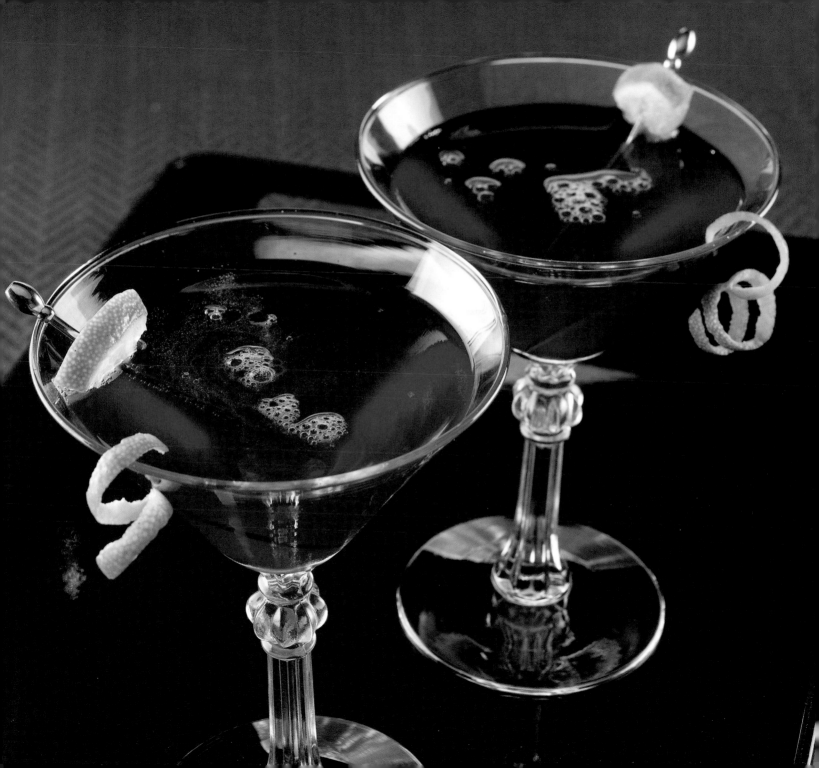

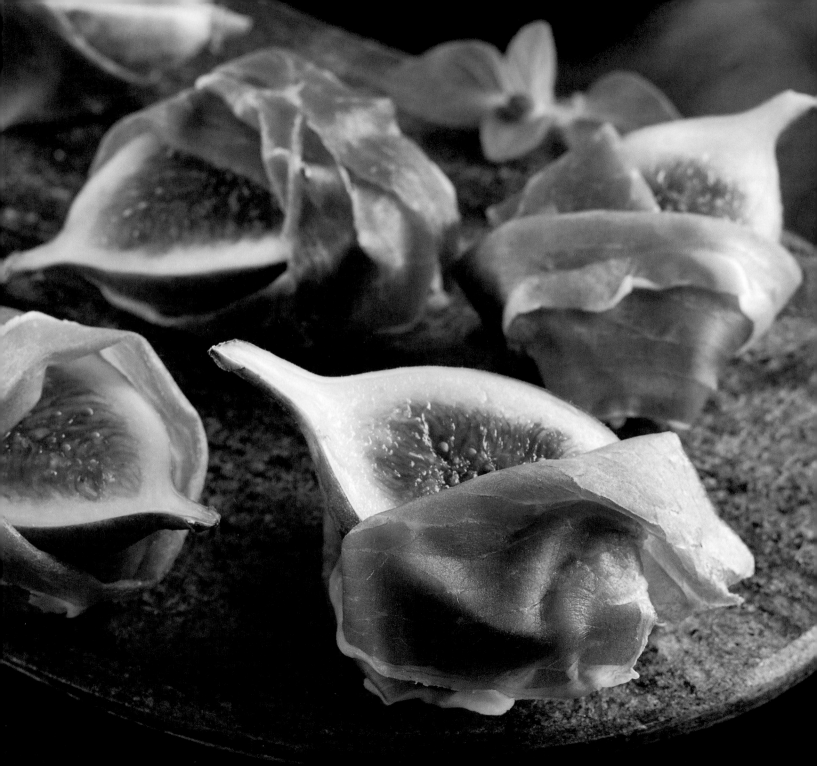

Prosciutto-Wrapped Figs or Melon

It's easy to increase the quantities of this simple appetizer if you're having a party. Make them just before you plan to eat. Wrapping the sweet-salty cured meat around the ripe juicy fruit takes just a few minutes.

Serves 2

1. Cut the figs in half or cut the melon into 8 wedges. Use a sharp knife to cut the rind from the melon.

2. Drizzle the fruit with the vinegar and sprinkle lightly with salt.

3. Cut the prosciutto slices in half lengthwise and wrap each slice around a piece of fruit.

4 ripe fresh figs or $^1/_2$ ripe honeydew or cantaloupe*

2 teaspoons (10 ml) balsamic or sherry vinegar

Sea salt

2 ounces (57 grams) prosciutto, cut into thin slices

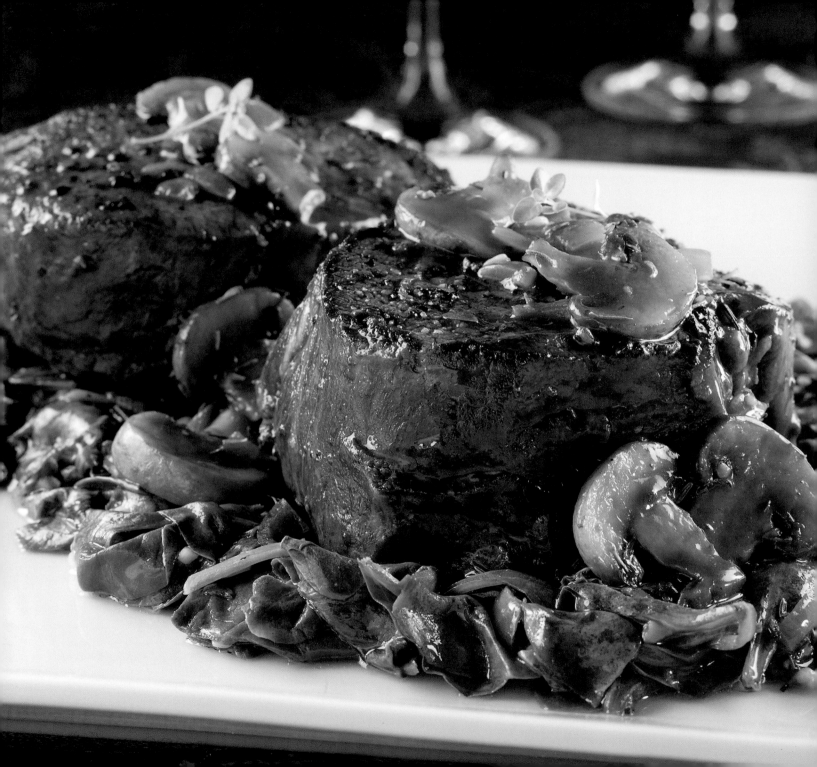

Filet Mignon with Sautéed Mushrooms

Lean filet mignon steaks are a delicious source of iron and carnitine—just right for a special dinner for two. Flavorful mushrooms add selenium. For a springtime variation, stir a half cup of blanched asparagus pieces into the sauce just before serving.

Serves 2

1. Sprinkle the steaks on both sides with salt and pepper. Heat 1 tablespoon (15 ml) oil in a large frying pan over medium-high heat. Add the steaks and cook for about 5 minutes per side for medium rare. Place steaks on a plate and keep warm.

2. Add the remaining tablespoon oil to the pan. Sauté the onion and garlic over medium heat for one minute. Add the mushrooms and oregano. Stir frequently until the mushrooms are browned and tender, 4 to 5 minutes.

3. Add the broth and vinegar and bring to a boil. Boil, stirring frequently, until the liquid has reduced slightly, 3 to 4 minutes. Season the mushrooms with salt and pepper to taste. Place the steaks on individual plates and spoon the mushrooms evenly over the steaks.

2 filet mignon steaks (each 4 to 6 ounces or 113 to 170 grams and about 1 inch thick)*

Salt

Freshly ground pepper

2 tablespoons (30 ml) olive oil, divided

3 tablespoon (15 ml) minced red onion

1 clove garlic, minced

3/4 pound (340 grams) mushrooms, thinly sliced*

1 teaspoon (5 ml) fresh oregano, or 1/4 teaspoon (1.25 ml) dried

1/4 cup (60 ml) beef or chicken broth

1 tablespoon (15 ml) balsamic vinegar

Mashed Sweet Potatoes or Yams with Yogurt and Lime

4 medium red sweet potatoes
(about 2 pounds or 908 grams)*

1/3 cup (80 ml)
plain whole-milk yogurt *

1 to 2 tablespoons
(15 to 30 ml) fresh lime juice

1/2 teaspoon (2.5 ml) salt

1/4 teaspoon (1.25 ml)
ground ginger

Freshly ground pepper

Use the red-fleshed sweet potatoes sometimes labeled "Garnet yams" (although they're not technically yams) for this sweet, tangy purée. It makes a delicious, healthy side dish for Thanksgiving, too.

Serves 4

1. Preheat the oven to 400°F (200°C).

2. Prick the potatoes all over with a fork and place in a baking pan. Bake until tender when pierced with a small sharp knife, about 50 minutes. Remove from the oven and let cool. When the potatoes are cool enough to handle, peel off the skin with the knife and discard. Place the sweet potatoes in a bowl.

3. Use a fork or a potato masher to coarsely mash the sweet potatoes with the remaining ingredients, adding pepper to taste. Before serving, reheat gently in a microwave or on a stove over low heat.

Wilted Spinach with Garlic

Spinach is truly a super vegetable; it's delicious, cooks in minutes, and goes well with just about everything. If you buy fresh spinach in a bunch, remove the leaves and place them in a large bowl of cold water. Swirl the leaves vigorously in the water to loosen any dirt, and rinse in several changes of cold water.

Serves 4

Heat the oil in a large frying pan over medium heat. Add the garlic and stir until fragrant but not browned, about 30 seconds. Add the spinach and stir until wilted, 1 to 2 minutes. Remove from the heat. Sprinkle with salt and pepper and serve immediately, with lemon wedges on the side for squeezing over the spinach.

2 tablespoons (30 ml) olive oil

2 cloves garlic, peeled and cut into thin slices

12 ounces (336 grams) spinach leaves, washed*

Sea salt

Freshly ground pepper

1 lemon, quartered

FERTILITY FACT:
Studies have shown that women who get most of their iron from nonmeat sources, like spinach, better their chances of getting pregnant compared to women who get most of their iron from meat.

Chocolate-Dipped Strawberry Bonbons

*4 ounces (170 grams)
bittersweet or semisweet
chocolate, chopped**

*6 large fresh strawberries with stems,
rinsed and patted dry**

*3 tablespoons (45 ml) chopped
pistachios**

Nothing says romance like strawberries and chocolate! Look for ripe, red strawberries and keep the leaves and stems on the strawberries for a pretty presentation, and have a few on hand for midnight snacks.

Serves 2; makes 6 strawberries

1. Line a baking sheet with wax paper. Place the chocolate in a heatproof bowl and set over a pan of barely simmering water. Stir frequently until the chocolate is melted and smooth.

2. Hold a strawberry by the stem end and dip it about three-fourths of the way into the chocolate, shaking the excess chocolate back into the bowl. Place it on the wax paper and repeat with the remaining strawberries.

3. Sprinkle the chocolate evenly with the pistachios. Place the baking sheet in the refrigerator until the chocolate is set, about 1 hour. Cover loosely with wax paper and store in the refrigerator for up to 1 day.

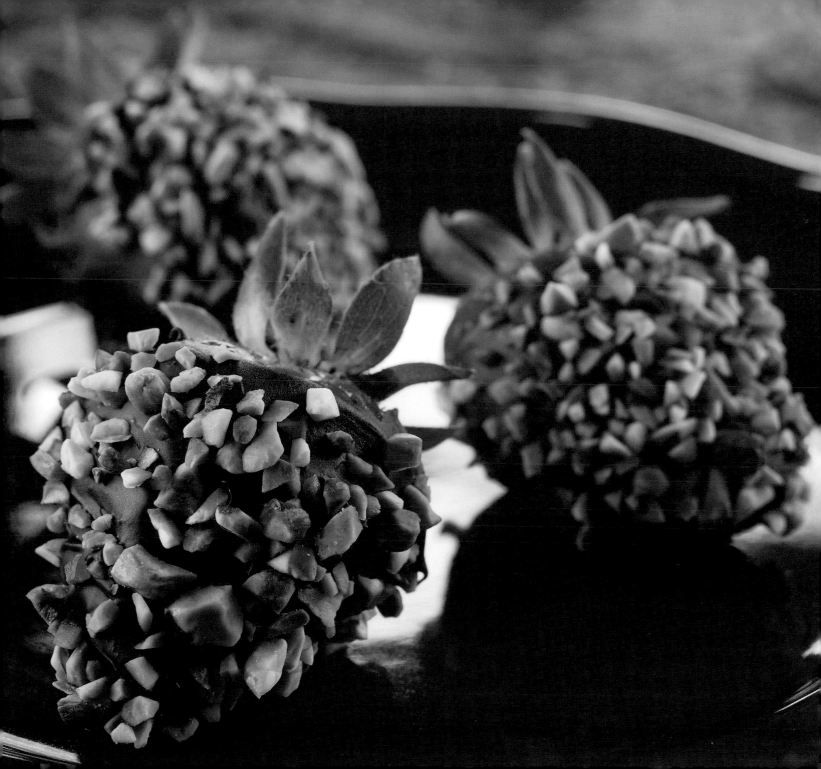

RESOURCES

ORGANIZATIONS AND WEB SITES

Conceive Magazine
Conceive Magazine and Conceive Online provide information and support for women at any stage of family building.
www.conceiveonline.com

American College of Obstetricians and Gynecologists (ACOG)
The Web site of this national organization of women's health care physicians provides patient information on all aspects of reproduction. **www.acog.org**

The American Fertility Association (AFA)
The AFA, a not-for-profit organization, provides information about infertility treatments, reproductive and sexual health, and family-building options, including surrogacy and adoption. **www.theafa.org**

American Society for Reproductive Medicine (ASRM)
An organization of specialists in reproductive medicine, the ASRM's Web site provides a wealth of information on infertility and its treatments. **www.asrm.org**

Centers for Disease Control and Prevention (CDC)
This government agency's site includes a preconception care–public health campaign urging women of reproductive age to get themselves healthy before becoming pregnant. A good resource for general and reproductive health information.
www.cdc.gov/ncbddd/preconception

Fertile Hope
This nonprofit organization is dedicated to helping cancer patients who are facing infertility after diagnosis and treatment.
www.fertilehope.org

Fertility LifeLines
An educational service provided by Serono, a pharmaceutical company. Callers to Fertility LifeLines speak with representatives, including nurse specialists, who can answer questions about fertility health concerns. **www.fertilitylifelines.com,**
1-866-LETS-TRY

The InterNational Council on Infertility Information Dissemination (INCIID)
INCIID (pronounced "inside") is a nonprofit organization that helps individuals and couples explore their family-building options. Scholarships are offered for families that need help financing treatment. **www.inciid.org**

This not-for-profit organization aims to improve the health of babies by educating the public about preconception and prenatal health and how to prevent birth defects, premature birth, and infant mortality. **www.marchofdimes.com**

RESOLVE: The National Infertility Association
Resolve is a nonprofit organization for men and women experiencing fertility disorders. The group has a network of chapters nationwide to promote reproductive health and raise awareness of infertility issues and family-building options. **www.resolve.org**

BOOKS
General Reproductive Health and Natural Conception

The Fertility Journal: A Day-by-Day Guide to Getting Pregnant
By Kim Hahn and the Editors of *Conceive Magazine* (Chronicle Books, 2008). A daily fill-in journal full of information about diet, exercise, lifestyle, and other factors that can influence conception.

Fertility Facts: Hundreds of Tips for Getting Pregnant
By Kim Hahn and the Editors of *Conceive Magazine*. (Chronicle Books, 2008). A compendium of hundreds of facts about reproduction, providing instant knowledge about diet, exercise, lifestyle, fertility treatments, and other factors that can influence conception.

The Everything Getting Pregnant Book: Professional, Reassuring Advice to Help You Conceive
By Robin Elise Weiss (Adams Media Corporation, 2004). Weiss, a certified childbirth educator, outlines the path to pregnancy, from going off birth control to considering fertility treatments.

Fertility and Conception: A Complete Guide to Getting Pregnant
By Zita West and Geoffrey Sher (DK Adult, 2003). A well-known British midwife (also author of *Plan to Get Pregnant*, DK Adult, 2008) with a holistic approach, West provides advice for couples who are newly trying to conceive as well as those who are experiencing problems. The book also discusses fertility treatment options, including IVF, neatly bridging the divide between conventional medicine and alternative treatments.

The Fertility Diet
By Jorge Chavarro, M.D., Walter C. Willett, M.D., and Patrick J. Skerrett (The McGraw-Hill Companies, Inc., 2007). Research results from the Nurses' Health Study at the Harvard School of Public Health indicate diet and lifestyle factors that boost ovulation and improve the chances of getting pregnant.

Preconception Plain & Simple: A Deliciously Smart and Sexy Guide in Preparing for Pregnancy
By Audrey Couto McClelland and Sharon K. Couto (Pinks and Blues Publishing, 2005). A fun book for couples just embarking on the fertility journey, this mother-daughter team of authors provides information on promoting fertility with foods, flowers, aromas, gemstones, and amulets. The idea is to follow the usual medical advice (provided), and then add a bit of romance and relaxation to conception.

Taking Charge of Your Fertility: The Definitive Guide to Natural Birth Control, Pregnancy Achievement, and Reproductive Health
By Toni Weschler, MPH (Collins Living, Tenth Anniversary Edition, 2006). This classic fertility tome explains how to use the fertility awareness method (FAM) to achieve or avoid pregnancy. By observing various fertility signs like morning temperature and cervical mucus, women learn to determine when they are ovulating.

Fertility Challenges

Conquering Infertility: Dr. Alice Domar's Mind/Body Guide to Enhancing Fertility and Coping with Infertility
By Alice D. Domar, Ph.D., and Alice Lesch Kelly (Penguin, 2004). Domar, an assistant professor of medicine at Harvard, gives women the tools they need to deal with the stress that can undermine fertility or arise from infertility. Topics include relaxation techniques such as yoga, meditation, journal writing, and guided imagery.

The Fertile Female: How the Power of Longing for a Child Can Save Your Life and Change the World
By Julia Indichova (Adell Press, 2007). Indichova, also author of *Inconceivable: A Woman's Triumph over Despair and Statistics* (Broadway, 2001), espouses a hopeful and empowering view of female fertility. The book includes nurturing advice as well as information on a fertility-friendly lifestyle and diet (including recipes).

I Am More Than My Infertility: 7 Proven Tools for Turning a Life Crisis into a Personal Breakthrough
By Marina Lombardo and Linda J. Parker (Seeds of Growth Press, 2007). Lombardo, *Conceive Magazine*'s "Emotionally Speaking" columnist, provides information and psychological support for women dealing with fertility challenges.

The Infertility Answer Book: The Complete Guide to Your Family-Building Choices with Fertility and Other Assisted Reproduction Technologies
By Brette McWhorter Sember (Sphinx Publishing, 2005). Sember, an attorney, answers the legal questions surrounding fertility treatments, third-party reproduction (donor egg, donor sperm, surrogates, and gestational carriers), and adoption. Along with medical advice, this book can help couples decide how to proceed when natural conception doesn't work.

The Infertility Cure: The Ancient Chinese Wellness Program for Getting Pregnant and Having Healthy Babies
By Randine Lewis (Little, Brown and Company, 2005). Lewis is a licensed acupuncturist and herbalist, and her book espouses Chinese medicine as an alternative to conventional western medicine and high-tech treatments.

100 Questions & Answers about Infertility
By John D. Gordon, M.D., and Michael DiMattina, M.D. (Jones and Bartlett Publishers, 2007). Two doctors answer the kinds of questions to which couples struggling with fertility problems want to know the answers.

Fertility Treatments, Including IVF

Conceptions & Misconceptions: The Informed Consumer's Guide through the Maze of In Vitro Fertilization and Other Assisted Reproduction Techniques
By Arthur L. Wisot, M.D., and David R. Meldrum, M.D. (Hartley and Marks Publishers, revised and expanded second edition, 2004). Two fertility specialists guide readers through the world of high-tech reproductive treatments, including tips for evaluating infertility clinics.

In Vitro Fertilization: The A.R.T.* of Making Babies
By Geoffrey Sher, M.D., Virginia Marriage Davis, RN, MN, and Jean Stoess, MA (Facts on File, third edition, 2005). A complete guide to IVF, including information for couples on how to determine whether they're eligible for treatment, how to select a good program, and an in-depth guide to how the technology works.

IVF & Ever After: The Emotional Needs of Families
By Nichola Bedos (Anshan Publishers, 2008) This book looks at IVF not from a medical perspective, but from a psychological one, using real-life stories and current research to examine the impact that this technology has on families and relationships. There are recommendations for how to manage the stress of treatment, and sections on raising a healthy family after IVF, including what to do with "extra" embryos, and how to tell a child about his or her conception.

What to Do When You Can't Get Pregnant: The Complete Guide to All the Technologies for Couples Facing Fertility Problems
By Daniel A. Potter, M.D., and Jennifer S. Hanin, M.D. (Da Capo Press, 2005). This book outlines all the reasons why couples may have trouble conceiving naturally, and then describes the gamut of low- and high-tech methods available to help. There's also a fascinating chapter on future and experimental technologies, such as stem-cell research and cloning.

INDEX

SUBJECT INDEX

RECIPE INDEX

A–B

C–D

TABLE OF EQUIVALENTS

LIQUID/DRY MEASUREMENTS

U.S.	Metric
1/4 teaspoon	1.25 milliliters
1/2 teaspoon	2.5 milliliters
1 teaspoon	5 milliliters
1 tablespoon (3 teaspoons)	15 milliliters
1 fluid ounce (2 tablespoons)	30 milliliters
1/4 cup	60 milliliters
1/3 cup	80 milliliters
1/2 cup	120 milliliters
3/4 cup	178 milliliters
1 cup	240 milliliters
1 pint (2 cups)	480 milliliters
1 quart (4 cups, 32 ounces)	960 milliliters
1 gallon (4 quarts)	3.84 liters
1 ounce (by weight)	28 grams
1 pound	448 grams
2.2 pounds	1 kilogram

LENGTHS

U.S.	Metric
1/8 inch	3 millimeters
1/4 inch	6 millimeters
1/2 inch	12 millimeters
1 inch	2.5 centimeters

OVEN TEMPERATURE

Fahrenheit	Celsius	Gas
250	120	1/2
275	140	1
300	150	2
325	160	3
350	180	4
375	190	5
400	200	6
425	220	7
450	230	8
475	240	9
500	260	10